CANYON RANCH

30 DAYS TO A BETTER BRAIN

CANYON RANCH

30 DAYS TO A BETTER BRAIN

A Groundbreaking Program for
Improving Your Memory, Concentration,
Mood, and Overall Well-Being

RICHARD CARMONA, MD, MPH, FACS

17th Surgeon General of the United States

ATRIA BOOKS

New York   London   Toronto   Sydney   New Delhi

ATRIA BOOKS
A Division of Simon & Schuster, Inc.
1230 Avenue of the Americas
New York, NY 10020

First Atria Books hardcover edition May 2014

ATRIA BOOKS and colophon are trademarks of Simon & Schuster, Inc.

For information about special discounts for bulk purchases, please contact Simon & Schuster Special Sales at 1-866-506-1949 or business@simonandschuster.com.

The Simon & Schuster Speakers Bureau can bring authors to your live event. For more information or to book an event contact the Simon & Schuster Speakers Bureau at 1-866-248-3049 or visit our website at www.simonspeakers.com.

Designed by Kyoko Watanabe
Interior artwork by Karen Morgenbesser
Jacket design by Jim Parsons, Canyon Ranch, Inc.

Manufactured in the United States of America

10   9   8   7   6   5   4   3   2   1

Library of Congress Cataloging-in-Publication Data
Carmona, Richard H.
Canyon Ranch 30 days to a better brain / by Richard Carmona, MD, MPH, FACS.
—First Atria hardcover edition.
pages cm
Includes bibliographical references and index.
1. Brain—Popular works. 2. Brain—Aging—Prevention—Popular works. 3. Mental efficiency—Popular works. 4. Self-care, Health—Popular works. I. Canyon Ranch. II. Title. III. Title: 30 days to a better brain. IV. Title: Canyon Ranch 30 days to a better brain.
QP376.C356 2014
612.8'2—dc23   2013008930

ISBN 978-1-4516-4380-0
ISBN 978-1-4516-4382-4 (ebook)

To all of our dedicated staff and professionals who have been, and continue to be, instrumental to the educational and therapeutic services that make Canyon Ranch exceptional. Their innovation in identifying and applying the best emerging science to our programs is a keystone to our success.

CONTENTS

PART THREE

Beyond Traditional Therapies

FOREWORD

Most people realize how precious their health is only when they are on the precipice of death. Usually it happens in a doctor's office or in an emergency room. But I've learned that it doesn't have to be this way, and I've dedicated my life to passing on this message.

I'm eighty-five years old, and I still work hard, feel good, and honestly enjoy life. But for my first fifty years I had a health profile I wouldn't wish on anyone. I was an asthmatic child who was told not to exercise. I was diagnosed with high blood pressure by the time I was twenty. By age twenty-four I suffered from duodenal ulcers, and by my mid-thirties I had diverticulitis and a hiatal hernia. In my forties my doctor told me I was starting to get osteoarthritis.

When my father died, I was nearing fifty, and besides all of my other health concerns, my weight was out of control. I asked my wife, Enid, to book me into a "fat farm," where I planned on staying for a week to help get my life back on track. That week turned into a month, and to this day I credit it with saving my life.

Within the first ten days, I had a remarkable transformation: I became the athlete I always dreamed of being, jogging at a rate that put me at the top of my age group. After three weeks, I begged Enid to come join me. "I've found what I want to do with the rest of my life," I told her. "We have to share this."

My miraculous reversal of health is the idea from which Canyon Ranch was born. Enid and I built our Tucson resort in 1978 as a place where we could live the healthy lives we wanted, and where we could share what we'd found with anyone who cared to come to us. The same philosophy that enabled me to change my life can help you change yours.

Today, more than thirty years and three properties later, people still think of Canyon Ranch as the ultimate health resort experience—a spa or retreat where they can get away from the stresses of life. The truth is, the services we offer are so much more than what most of our first-time guests ever imagine. Every year, thousands of people come to our Canyon Ranch locations for many different, highly personal reasons. Some come to recharge themselves in our extraordinary natural settings; others travel to improve their health or focus on their diet or get back into an exercise routine. Yet the reasons that bring them to us really aren't important. What we concentrate on are the advances guests can make while they are here, because we know that what we offer can effect changes that will last a lifetime.

Everyone who works with us at Canyon Ranch is intensely passionate about what they do. Together, we've created a wellness revolution based on a preventive, integrative approach. All of our practitioners teach a singular message: you can participate actively in your health and well-being, reaping the rewards now and for years to come. Our job is to figure out where each guest needs to make a change, using an extensive list of modalities ranging from traditional medicine to alternative healing, and every aspect of lifestyle enhancement. This is especially effective when it comes to maximizing the brain's potential.

We've created this exciting new book in order to let you experience right in your own home everything that Canyon Ranch has to offer. Your journey to better brain health begins with embracing the Canyon Ranch philosophy, which is based on four spheres of well-being:

- The Physical: Am I taking care of my body?
- The Mental: Am I actively engaged in learning?
- The Emotional: Am I working toward balance?
- The Spiritual: Am I connected to something outside myself?

I'm so pleased that you've begun your journey to better brain health with us. Over the next thirty days you'll see for yourself how all these seemingly disparate ideas fit together in order for you to become the very best that you can be. You'll learn that by just making small changes to your lifestyle you can improve your mood, memory, and cognition, as well as your overall health. And hopefully, we will inspire you to recognize the power of possibility in your own life.

MEL ZUCKERMAN, COFOUNDER OF CANYON RANCH
TUCSON, ARIZONA

AUTHOR'S NOTE

My relationship with Canyon Ranch first began when I moved to Tucson twenty-nine years ago. Back then, Canyon Ranch was a relatively new entity, a few years old and struggling to survive. I immediately identified with Mel and Enid's vision for creating a sanctuary for pursuing health and wellness, because I had learned on my own personal journey the importance of preventive care.

I was born in New York City to an immigrant family who struggled to provide for their children. I grew up in Harlem. We were poor, even homeless for a while. I was a truant, ran the streets, and eventually enlisted in the army at seventeen years old. Once in the army, I got my high school equivalency diploma and thrived in a community based on structure. I went into the infantry, then on to airborne and the U.S. Army Special Forces during the Vietnam War. I thought I was going to make a career in the military, but my Special Forces teammates and my high school counselors encouraged me to go to college.

When I returned to New York I enrolled in Bronx Community College in a program for Vietnam veterans and eventually transferred to the City University of New York, then finished college in California. While I was in school I held lots of different jobs, all of which put me in a position to help others. I've been a police officer, ocean lifeguard, paramedic, registered nurse, and physician's assistant. After graduation, I went to University of California, San Francisco, School of Medicine, and then trained as a general vascular surgeon with a subspecialty in trauma, burns, and critical care. I was recruited to Tucson and the University of Arizona Medical Center to start the first certified trauma care system in Arizona. Although I thought I'd be in Tucson only a couple of years, I ended up staying just about my whole adult life.

Throughout these experiences, I realized that most of what I was treating was preventable. I began to transition from clinical care into public health, where I could begin to make a difference in promoting the things we can do to prevent disease and pursue optimal health and wellness. I decided to go to night school at the University of Arizona, where I was a professor, and I received my master's degree in Public Health Policy and Administration. During that time I transitioned to running a public hospital and health system. Then in 2002 I was nominated to be surgeon general of the United States and was confirmed unanimously by the U.S. Senate. I served in that position for four years, which is the statutory term. It's also a uniformed position: I had the rank of vice admiral and was the leader of the United States Public Health Service Commissioned Corps. The job description of the surgeon general is to protect, promote, and advance the health, safety, and security of the nation.

When I arrived in Tucson in 1985, I built a house at Canyon Ranch Estates, which is where I raised my family. Over the years I would be invited to the ranch every once in a while to give a lecture. I appreciated and enjoyed living the lifestyle that Canyon Ranch preached, which is about optimal health and wellness. Mel and Enid and their partner Jerry Cohen became good friends of mine because they appreciated the way I conducted my life: I eat healthy, most of the time, and I exercise on a regular basis. When I left the office of the surgeon general, I was offered many different positions, both academic and in the business world, but the one that intrigued me the most was right here at home. Mel and Jerry asked me to be a vice chairman of the organization and also to establish and lead the Canyon Ranch Institute, of which the goal is to deliver the content of Canyon Ranch to underserved communities throughout the world. Six years later, I continue to love what I do every single day.

One of the things I've noticed over the years—both as a citizen trying to stay healthy and in all the roles I've had over several decades, including being a nurse, a paramedic, and a physician—is that while people are experiencing longer and healthier lives, our bodies are sometimes outliving our minds. Physicians and therapists are treating more cognitive decline than ever before, whether it's Alzheimer's disease, dementia, or other issues related to brain health. So the idea struck me that the medical community spends an inordinate amount of time trying to teach people to eat healthy and exercise and take care of the body, but is doing relatively little to preserve cognitive health. As I looked at all my experiences, it became apparent that with a growing and aging population, we need to address preventing cognitive decline as it is related to physical aging. Whether I was treating people with head injuries, taking care of aging seniors, or helping victims of strokes, I knew that there was more we could be doing. I also knew that even if there are already signs of an aging brain, we are now able to slow down and, in some disease states, maybe even avert some of the expected cognitive decline by making simple lifestyle alterations through nutrition, physical activity, and more.

Next, I challenged the Canyon Ranch medical and therapeutic teams in all of our locations to put together a plan and bring a Canyon Ranch approach to the issue of brain health. When we looked at the science, it was very clear that there's a lot we can do to prevent cognitive decline. And interestingly, it turns out that many of the things that we're doing to maintain a healthy body are also good for the brain.

I wanted to create a truly integrative approach. At Canyon Ranch, we deal with issues of mind, body, and spirit to pursue optimal health and wellness. So I asked the experts to formulate a program that can help readers like you to preserve and/or enhance cognitive function so that as you physically age you can minimize or prevent cognitive decline. That's what the book is all about—how to make the best choices every day in order to improve your physical ability and to enhance or preserve your cognitive functions as you age. Even if you're in your seventies, eighties, or nineties, you can still learn; you can still teach an old dog new tricks!

This book reflects the intellectual knowledge of all our practitioners, who cover many diverse areas of wellness, because each of those areas has an impact on your cognitive health. Just by reading this book you'll be learning from the best in traditional medicine, complementary and alternative medicine, behavioral science, exercise physiology, and nutrition. And hopefully, I'll meet you at one of our properties one day so that you can share your success story with me.

RICHARD CARMONA, MD, MPH, FACS,
SEVENTEENTH SURGEON GENERAL OF THE UNITED STATES
TUCSON, ARIZONA

INTRODUCTION

According to the 2011 MetLife Foundation Alzheimer's Survey, American adults are just as concerned about their brain and the possibility of living out their later years with dementia or Alzheimer's disease as they are worried about developing cancer. This may be due to the fact that many cancers are seen as treatable, while a loss of cognitive function seems irreversible. It's also possible that the underlying preoccupation with a failing brain uncovers a larger problem—many of us are simply uncomfortable with aging, especially as we watch our older relatives in their final days. Many of our loved ones unfortunately suffered with cognitive loss after leading sedentary lives or never taking care of their health.

It's very likely that we will live longer than our parents and grandparents. And while we are living longer, we've come to expect that we can also live younger. In order to do that, we need to have strong, agile minds that can keep up with and help maintain strong bodies. But while we may think we're doing all we can—or at least understand what we should do—to help keep our bodies healthy, many of us don't know where to begin when it comes to taking care of our brains.

Until quite recently, there wasn't much advice any respectable doctor or therapist could offer that would make dramatic improvements in cognition—that is, your memory, attention, and mood. However, the latest technological advances in medical imaging have given us a real window into the workings of the brain, and every day we are learning more about exactly how the brain functions, where problems arise, and what we can do to effectively halt and possibly reverse damage and dysfunction. What's more, we now know that the brain can continue to change and grow as we get older, making the promise of maintaining—and even enhancing—cognitive abilities as well as overall brain health a reality.

At Canyon Ranch, we aim to inspire in each person a commitment to healthy living and to provide the tools and knowledge to turn intentions into reality. Along this path, we've identified many simple lifestyle choices that each of us can make to ensure a better, younger brain now, and for years to come. Our specialists focus on the many different, yet equally critical, components of brain health. Their findings are verified by the most up-to-date research available and are framed by our unique philosophy, which combines best practices in wellness, fitness, traditional and alternative medicine, nutritional support, and spiritual guidance. Together, this integrated and holistic approach offers the greatest opportunity to improve brain function and prevent decline. This is especially true if you are not yet experiencing any of the signs or symptoms of an aging brain; just as with any other aspect of your health, you'll reap the greatest benefits from a program based on prevention.

The benefits of improving your brain health are many:

- Better memory
- Better mood
- Better sleep
- Faster and more accurate thinking
- Greater efficiency
- Improved balance
- Improved overall health
- Increased energy
- Quicker reactions and reflexes
- Safer driving
- Self-confidence
- Sharper listening

Spend the Next 30 Days at Canyon Ranch

People come to Canyon Ranch from all over the world to increase their longevity and well-being. Now imagine that you are one of these people, but instead of coming for a few days, you'll be here for a month. You'll leave the distractions of your everyday life behind and focus completely and deeply on improving your brain health. You'll have unlimited access to our vast array of programs and specialists. You'll be pampered and restored, ready to face your world again. Best of all, you'll notice that you're calmer, more relaxed, and thinking and feeling better than ever before.

The thirty-day program in this book allows you to investigate all the components that can improve brain health and to see how they fit together to promote, reverse, and—most important—prevent problems. Our staff of doctors, nurses, health professionals, and life management consultants have all worked together to create a comprehensive brain health program that is based on lifestyle modification—the small changes you can make to the way you live your life that will help you take better care of your brain. In fact, many of the things you may be currently doing, such as exercising and maintaining a proper weight through good nutrition, also turn out to be the foundations for improving brain health. At the end of the program, you'll have the language—the health literacy—to continue this conversation with your health care provider so that you can stay with this program and work together in order to make good decisions about your health and medical care.

How This Book Works

Part One explores the many different factors that affect brain health. It begins with an overview of the brain, including its unique structure and function. The information in this book is completely up-to-date and is presented so clearly that you'll easily master the science, and we know that the only way to create lasting and sustainable behavioral change is to be able to take ownership of the information and apply what you've learned to your life.

You'll learn how normal aging changes the brain's physical and mental functioning, and why it is the most common culprit in beginning the spiral of cognitive decline. Next, you'll learn how your unique genetic makeup and current health status may be aging your brain prematurely; it turns out that the full spectrum of chronic diseases and mild annoyances can all affect the way you think. You'll come to understand how your emotional life affects your mood as well as your memory, and you'll learn how you can master the best ways to deal with stress, depression, and addiction. You'll also be introduced to the many different ways that a toxic environment can affect your thinking as well as other brain functions. Last, you'll discover why you may not be sleeping and what you can do to restore and reset your brain each night.

Part Two presents the thirty-day brain health program. First, you'll learn exactly what you need to eat to promote brain health. Each week focuses on different nutrients and includes foods that are rich in antioxidants, healthy fats, and more. You'll also follow along with our signature exercise programs, which promote cardiovascular fitness, the best type of exercise for brain health. There are dozens of suggested workouts that increase in difficulty as you master them throughout the month. Last, you'll learn how to remove stress from your life and let in spirituality through various meditation practices, all of which are beneficial to brain health. By the end of the month, you'll be able to quantify how much better you think, look, and feel.

Part Three highlights additional options to improve your brain function, focusing on some of the many traditional and alternative therapies that we offer at Canyon Ranch. You may realize that you require further medical testing or are interested in exploring a full brain-health assessment, and you'll have a list of medical and cognitive tests to discuss with your doctor. There is a detailed list of supplements you might want to consider based on your current health status, and there are delicious and easy recipes that incorporate the best foods for your brain. You'll also learn the ways in which acupuncture and energy healing therapies can help balance your brain. You'll come to understand why it is necessary to always maintain a high level of curiosity, and you'll be able to choose among a myriad of activities that will keep you socially engaged as well as enhance your cognitive functioning, from computer games to adult education and more. By the end of the book, you'll have developed a detailed plan that covers exactly what you can do every day to support your brain's health. We like to think of it as a perfect day at the ranch, and we hope that you will, too.

Only you have the power to make the necessary changes in your life and start taking control of your health. Together, we can create a rich and engaged life full of good decisions that positively affect your well-being, both of the body and of the brain.

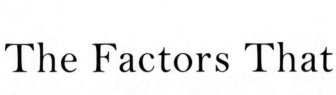

PART ONE

The Factors That Affect Brain Health

Chapter 1

―――――

HOW THE BRAIN WORKS

If you've been taking your brain for granted, you're not alone. Most people assume their brain is working just as well as ever, even as they get older. But the reality can be far different.

The brain is a highly responsive organ that is involved in every internal function of the body, from regulating metabolism to controlling balance and coordination to governing our sex lives and, of course, all the activities associated with the senses and the mind, particularly mood and memory. The brain's functioning is central to the concept of the *mind-body connection,* the way the body's health responds to our thoughts, feelings, and actions. This connection illustrates how our emotional life can both positively and negatively affect our physical health and how our physical health can affect our mood and cognition. The truth is that the brain and the rest of the body are one unit of health; the brain is affected by many of the same diseases and conditions that distress our physical health. At the same time, it is also susceptible to aging and even injury.

Monitoring the brain's health is not always as obvious or easy as evaluating changes to the rest of the body. Many of us notice the aches and pains as well as the signs and symptoms of physical aging. You know when you've put on weight even though your diet hasn't changed, and you can tell when your joints hurt more than they did last year. But you might not notice that your thinking has slowed down or your attention is not sharp or your moods or anxiety levels have changed. This is mostly due to the fact that the brain is hidden from our view; we can't see it aging as clearly as we can see the gray hairs coming in or our jawline slackening.

The brain also has enormous *biological reserve,* the extensive backup plan to keep all aspects of your health—physical as well as emotional—running smoothly. This reserve allows the body to continue functioning as we age and gives us a false sense of security in terms of our cognition; we actually can get by with substantial loss of brain function without realizing that changes have occurred. This reserve makes it very difficult to recognize if there has been a slowing in our mental capacity until there is a significant change. Yet unfortunately, once you do notice, it means that the underlying problem that has caused this change has been going on for a very long time.

The good news is that just like the rest of your body, your brain can get better. By starting a program based on improving your brain health now, you can begin to recognize subtle changes and have the opportunities to enhance your brain's capabilities so that it can serve you well now and for years to come. Science has only just recently confirmed what we at Canyon Ranch have believed all along: your lifestyle can influence your health. This research has blossomed into a new field called *epigenetics,* which suggests that it is possible to alter one's genetic destiny by changing nongenetic factors—such as lifestyle choices. These specific behaviors can actually cause a person's genes to turn on or off without changing the underlying DNA sequencing. In other words, to a very large extent, you are in control of your own health. And nowhere is this more exciting to consider than in terms of your brain's potential.

This book is meant to set you on the path to better brain health. We believe that this is the highest pursuit in wellness that you can become engaged with, because you really can't be healthy without a healthy brain. And it terms of your longevity, your brain's functioning is as important as that of any other organ in your body, including your heart.

We all hope for and have come to expect to live long lives. A hundred years ago, the average person could expect to live between forty-nine and fifty-one years. Today if you are in good health, it's reasonable to assume that you will live well into your eighties and even beyond. Medical technology is one of the underlying reasons for this enormous increase: we have easy access to a host of treatments and procedures that can keep our internal organs and bone structure from failing. However, our ability to increase longevity has not fully addressed many of the problems associated with an aging brain. The truth is, half of the people who reach eighty-five years of age will have some form of dementia or cognitive dysfunction. This knowledge alone is exactly why improving brain health is so critical: we want not only to maintain a vibrant, healthy body for years to come but for those years to be of the highest quality. And the only way to ensure that is by maintaining—or even enhancing—a vibrant, healthy brain. By doing so, you'll increase your capacity to live life to its fullest every day.

Understanding Your Brain

The brain is a complex and sophisticated organ, and to work on improving its health, it's important to understand both its structure and how it functions. On the smallest scale the brain is made of 100 billion individual *neurons,* or brain cells. Neurons are the electrically excitable cells that process and transmit information to each other through *neurotransmitters,* or brain chemicals. Together, these neurons and neurotransmitters form a specialized network that governs how we feel and think.

Each neuron is composed of a cell body, dendrites, and one axon. More than 150 different types of neurons exist, so they are some of the most diverse cells in the human body. Dendrites and axons are thin structures that branch off the neuronal cell body. Each cell body is surrounded by multiple dendrites, but never more than one axon. In simplest terms, one neuron's dendrite connects to another's axon, but the two do not completely touch. With 100 billion neurons, this allows for 100 trillion connections between them. Each connection creates a *synapse,* the place where the chemical and electrical signals of the brain are sent and received.

The axon is protected by a *myelin sheath,* an insulation barrier much like the material surrounding an electrical wire. The myelin sheath helps the axon hold on to its chemical message until it's delivered to the next cell.

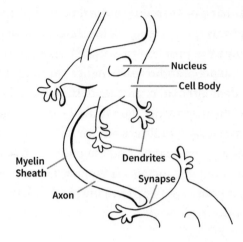

A NEURON OR BRAIN CELL

The brain's function is measured by how well your neuronal network is working: Are the neurons hooked up to each other in the right way? Are they making the same or new connections? Are there any short circuits? And most important, how quickly can they transfer information? This transmission is referred to as *brain processing speed.* Damage to any part of this system limits or prevents the neuronal message from transferring from one cell to the next. Speed, then, is important in the sense that it is necessary for maintaining the information traveling through the axon so that it can be relayed to the next neuron. A normal brain responds to stimuli at a speed of at least one-third of a second. Typically, we lose seven to ten milliseconds of brain speed per decade from age twenty on. The difference between a resourceful mind and senility is only one hundred milliseconds. When this loss occurs, the neurons can no longer fire their chemical messages fast enough to affect the actions they were governing. That is why as we age we move more slowly, misjudge distances, and make mistakes.

This loss of brain speed is one of the main causes of *mild cognitive impairment,* or MCI. People generally start to see these declines when they reach their seventies, yet they can begin to notice changes in their thinking in their forties. By the age of forty, 25 to 50 percent of Americans are already affected by MCI, even though less than 1 percent will show any symptoms. In an aging brain, the neurons themselves, the quality and quantity of their neurotransmitters, or the neuronal connections can be altered, and thereby affect your brain's health. Brain cells die off, or their connections become broken, making it more difficult to retrieve stored information, or what we refer to as memories.

As we get older, we think that we are becoming more forgetful. The truth is that we don't actually lose memories; instead, we lose the capacity and the speed required for retrieving them. The goal, then, for enhancing brain health is to maintain and improve these neurons, as well as their connections, for as long as possible, because an efficient brain is a smarter brain.

This strategy is particularly true when it comes to those myelin sheaths surrounding the axons. These protective coverings can disintegrate, and plaques made up of sticky proteins called *beta-amyloid* can build up on them. Or these axonal connections become entangled with accumulations of other proteins. Both of these scenarios are present in the diagnosis of Alzheimer's disease, the most invasive form of dementia.

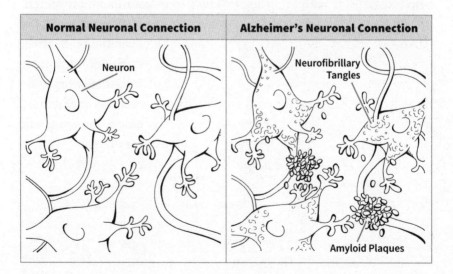

THE REGIONS OF THE BRAIN

Depending on where neurons are located in the brain, their function changes. For example, there are *sensory neurons* that respond to touch, sound, light, smell, and taste. *Motor neurons* receive signals from the brain and spinal cord, causing muscle movement. Each neuronal network creates distinct *lobes,* or regions of the brain, and each is responsible for different aspects of our mental, physical, and cognitive health. However, these brain regions are often responsible for multiple tasks, and their functions often overlap.

The brain is composed of three distinct parts: the cerebrum, the brain stem, and the cerebellum. The *cerebrum,* or forebrain, is the largest part of the brain. It is covered by the *cerebral cortex.* This is the collection of folded bulges—known as gray matter—that comes to mind when we think about the brain. These bulges increase the brain's surface area and enable us to fit a great volume into a small area. Together, the cerebral cortex and the cerebrum play a key role in memory, attention, awareness, thought, language, and consciousness.

The next region of the brain is the *cerebellum.* It is a ball of tissue below and behind the cerebrum that decodes sensory information and integrates it with your body's muscles to coordinate movement. Finally, the *brain stem* links the brain to the spinal cord. It controls bodily functions such as heart rate, blood pressure, and breathing.

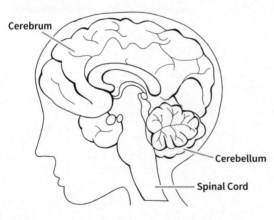

REGIONS OF THE BRAIN

Analyzing the Cerebrum

The cerebrum is divided into two hemispheres, left and right, that are linked by a thick band of nerve fibers called the *corpus callosum*. Messages to and from one side of the body are usually handled by the opposite side of the brain, meaning the left hemisphere controls the right side of the body.

The hemispheres are identical in that they contain the same types of lobes. Each hemisphere is further divided into four lobes, all of which create and retrieve memories. From the descriptions below, you can see how their functions often overlap:

- The frontal lobes control thinking, planning, organizing, problem solving, short-term memory, and movement.
- The parietal lobes interpret sensory information, such as taste, temperature, and touch.
- The occipital lobes process visual information and link that information with memory.
- The temporal lobes process smell, taste, and sound. They also play a role in memory storage.

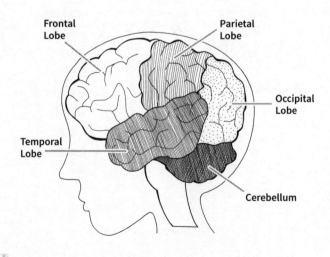

LOBES OF THE BRAIN

Within the middle region of the cerebrum lie several small structures that form the *limbic system,* which is involved in many of our
emotions and motivations, including fear, anger, and pleasure. Certain
structures of the limbic system are involved in creating and maintaining
memory.

Amygdala: This is located in the temporal lobe and is responsible for determining how memories are stored and where the
memories are stored in the brain. It is thought that this determination is based on the emotional response an event invokes.

Hippocampus: This is where short-term memories are stored
before they are moved to the appropriate lobes of the cerebrum,
and it organizes how memories are retrieved when necessary.
Damage to this area of the brain may result in an inability to
form new memories; the hippocampus is one of the primary
areas of the brain affected by Alzheimer's disease.

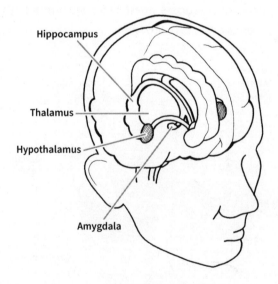

Hippocampus

Thalamus

Hypothalamus

Amygdala

THE LIMBIC SYSTEM

Hypothalamus: This controls emotions, eating, and sleeping. About the size of a pearl, this structure, in concert with the pituitary gland, indirectly affects adrenaline production when needed for the control of emotions. Adrenaline is a hormone involved in making you feel exhilarated, angry, or unhappy, as well as activating the fight-or-flight response.

Thalamus: This transfers messages from the spinal cord to other areas within the hemisphere.

AN AGING BRAIN IS A SMALLER BRAIN

Healthy brains can maintain their original structure, but an aging brain is drier and smaller than a young brain. By the time you reach your seventies, the brain will have shrunk about 10 percent and will look more wrinkled than a younger version. The change in the size of your brain doesn't cause pain, and you can't feel it occur. And because the brain is encased in the skull, you can't see these changes, either.

When Does Decline Begin?

According to the Baltimore Longitudinal Study of Aging, adults reach their physical peak somewhere between ages twenty-eight and thirty-two. Beyond that, your brain will age either at the same rate as the rest of your body or faster or slower. Damage or dysfunction in any one of the regions ages the brain, sometimes faster than your chronological age. This means that a head injury—even one sustained when you were younger—can affect your thinking later in life, aging your brain faster than the rest of your body.

One way to identify a prematurely aging brain is through your sense of smell. Losing it is one of the first signs that there is a problem with the brain and can predict memory loss. Sense of smell declines because the type of cells in the nasal cavity of the brain (known as *granule cells*) are the same type as the cells in the hippocampus, where short-term memories reside, and both these cells age at the same rate.

The entire brain is surrounded by blood vessels that continuously nourish it and by *cerebrospinal fluid,* which bathes, protects, and cushions it. The *ventricles,* the areas beneath and around the brain, produce a bath of cerebrospinal fluid that moves all the way around the outside of the brain and the spinal cord. As the brain shrinks, the ventricles enlarge by filling the void with fluid. Enlarged ventricles may be an indication of brain shrinkage and are a common finding in those with dementia.

THE BASICS OF BRAIN CHEMISTRY

The structure of the brain tells only half the story; the rest of brain health is related to how the brain functions. The *neurotransmitters,* the chemical messengers sent between the neurons, are created in the cell body and transported from the axon into a synapse, where they bind to chemical receptors located in the dendrites. You can think of a neurotransmitter as a key and a receptor as a lock: together, they open the door. We also know that the same type of key can be used to open many different types of locks, and some locks may accept a number of similar keys. The effect on the target neuron—what happens once the door is opened—is determined not by the source neuron or by the neurotransmitter but by the type of receptor that is activated. In a healthy brain, the acceptance of these neurotransmitters occurs in a smooth, rhythmic flow. However, the delivery or production of these brain chemicals can become unbalanced and dysfunctional, affecting our health as well as our mood, memory, and attention.

Scientists are still identifying all of the neurotransmitters, and we currently know of at least fifty different types. The ones that we know the most about include:

Acetylcholine: Plays a very important role in memory. It conducts sensory input signals and stimulates muscular movement.

Adrenaline: Also referred to as epinephrine. It increases heart rate, sharpens reflexes, constricts blood vessels, dilates air passages, and participates in the way we respond to stressful situations, including the fight-or-flight response.

Dopamine: Helps control the brain's reward and pleasure centers. It enables us to not only see rewards but take action to move toward them. Dopamine also helps regulate movement and emotional responses.

Gamma-Aminobutyric Acid (GABA): An amino acid that acts as a neurotransmitter. It has a calming effect on the brain, blocking nerve impulses. Without GABA, nerve cells fire too often and too easily. Anxiety disorders such as panic attacks, seizure ailments, and other conditions, including cognitive impairment, are all related to low GABA activity.

Noradrenaline (Norepinephrine): Has a stimulating effect, fosters alertness, and plays an important role in long-term memory and learning. Optimal levels of this neurotransmitter can stimulate a sense of well-being, yet an excess can fuel fear and anxiety.

Serotonin: Is involved in about one quarter of all our biological processes. Serotonin has been shown to play a role in modifying mood, particularly with depression.

AN AGING BRAIN CAN AFFECT YOUR LIFE

When your brain ages significantly, you may begin to feel or act differently. Some people notice that they feel tired all the time, either because their sleep is disturbed or because they are simply always fatigued. Others begin to feel more anxious or less connected to friends and family, and become unmotivated—and sometimes mentally unable— to leave the home. You might feel more forgetful or lack the ability or desire to plan, execute, or have abstract thoughts. Your attention may wander, along with your balance or hand-eye coordination. You may notice that things you used to be able to do quickly are taking longer, including your reaction time, ability to solve problems, or facility in learning new tasks.

Changes in the brain can affect your weight, your bone density, and your muscular control. What's more, when you become withdrawn and don't want to leave your home, you won't get enough exercise, and your muscles will atrophy. Simply put, an aging brain can make you look and feel much older than your chronological age.

Your brain's health exists on a spectrum. At one end is fully functioning activity—what we call a youthful brain. MCI is located along the arc, and unless your brain's health is shored up, it will continue to diminish until full dementia occurs. Dementia is defined as a loss of brain function that significantly affects memory, thinking, language, judgment, and behavior. The farthest point on the spectrum is where Alzheimer's disease (AD) can reside. Alzheimer's disease is actually a type of dementia and is an incredibly debilitating condition that is directly connected to an aging brain.

However, we can prevent and even delay the cognitive impairment that leads to AD. The goal of this book is to teach you how to delay MCI so that it won't change your life until you are in your nineties instead of your seventies. If we can address the earliest, mildest losses of cognitive function, you'll have the best opportunity to make a positive difference in how you enjoy the rest of your life.

THE DIFFERENCES BETWEEN DEMENTIA AND ALZHEIMER'S DISEASE

We all experience "brain blips" from time to time: forgetting where we put eyeglasses, overlooking items on a shopping list, or even walking into a room and losing track of why we are there. But at what point is misplacing your car keys considered a hallmark of old age or something worse? And are brain blips the first sign of an aging brain?

Some changes in brain function occur as a part of natural aging. For example, at age sixty, as compared to twenty, it may take a little longer to think on your feet and remember something. When these blips occur with great frequency, you may be experiencing the neurological condition called *mild cognitive impairment*. When this happens, lapses in finding words and recalling names are common, along with other difficulties that can include failing to remember appointments or losing one's train of thought in the middle of a conversation. Though MCI is not as severe as full-blown Alzheimer's disease, many believe it is the beginning of a spectrum that leads to other forms of dementia. The good news is that this type of impairment can, in most cases, be rectified by following a health plan like the one outlined in this book.

However, people with Alzheimer's disease will exhibit certain classic features or behaviors that are caused by the disease and become more pronounced as the disease progresses. We call these changes the Four As of Alzheimer's, and they are directly related to the lobes of the brain where aging or damage has occurred.

Amnesia: The inability to use or retain memory, including short-term and long-term memory. True amnesia may lead someone to confusion, where the person suffering repeats questions such as "Where am I?" "Who are you?" Amnesia occurs when there is damage to the frontal lobes.

Agnosia: The inability to recognize or deal with common objects and/or people. Those suffering with agnosia may become lost even in a very familiar place. They may confuse common household items, store belongings in seemingly strange places (i.e., putting away a frying pan in the freezer), and confuse even the closest family members. This process is associated with increased damage to the frontal lobes, the occipital lobes, and the temporal lobes.

Aphasia: The inability to use or understand language. Aphasia begins with the sufferer using the wrong word or losing his or her train of thought, or providing a description of an object or place because he or she can't access the right word. Aphasia is associated with damage to the temporal and frontal lobes.

Apraxia: The inability to use or coordinate purposeful muscle movement.

In the early stages of apraxia, the sufferer may reach for an item and miss it. Eventually balance becomes affected, leading to an increase in the risk of falls and injury. Apraxia is linked to damage to the parietal lobes, the cerebral cortex, and the occipital lobes.

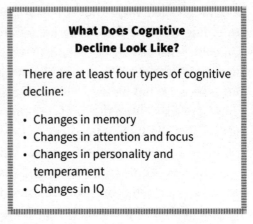

What Does Cognitive Decline Look Like?

There are at least four types of cognitive decline:

- Changes in memory
- Changes in attention and focus
- Changes in personality and temperament
- Changes in IQ

How Memory Works

Memories are the functional building blocks of the brain—the brain literally grows as it is exposed to new stimuli, and records that information as memories. Memory is the process of storage and retrieval of information and experience and resides in vast chains of brain cells—neuronal networks—rather than a single brain cell. Each cell holds only a portion of information, and you need to be able to connect these cells to access memories. Many functions of the brain are really just complex memory processes, which are regularly reworked because of new learning and emotional growth. But if we cannot receive information we cannot process it or store it.

Brain processing speed affects the way you retrieve your memories. Again, it's not really that you lose memory; it's just that the time it takes to retrieve the memory increases and the extent to which we can retrieve decreases. If you have fewer neuronal connections, you have limited options in terms of how you retrieve memories.

There are many ways to categorize memory, including short-term and long-term memory, as well as memories related to your senses.

Long-Term Memory: When you hear a certain song from your teenage years, it may take you back to your senior prom. Or a certain smell can take you back to your mother's kitchen. These are long-term memories, and they demonstrate that there are many tools your brain can use to store and remember data. For example, when you lose your keys (as we all do), most of us think of where we saw them last. But if you chose a different trigger, like the feeling of the key in your hand, you might be able to call on the memory differently.

Verbal/Auditory Memory: The ability to absorb and retain verbally presented information. Verbal memories are thought to be stored in the temporal lobes. Roughly 20 percent of learners have high auditory skills, and these people are able to compartmentalize complex material, but are less confident in their own memory.

Visual Memory: The ability to absorb and retain information such as colors, shapes, designs, pictures, and symbols. The occipital lobes are responsible for this type of visual training. The

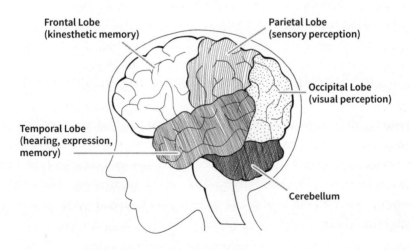

MEMORY IS STORED
WITHIN THE BRAIN'S LOBES

majority of people (more than 65 percent) learn through visual memory. These are the people who typically learn quickly and are able to see the "big picture" of life.

Kinesthetic Memory: Kinesthetic memories are based on your physical relationship to the world. They help keyboard users type rapidly without having to look at the keys, just as musicians can play their instruments without consciously having to think about the necessary movements. And this kind of memory can help people to find something again, by remembering the location where they put it.

Immediate Memory: Lasting only thirty seconds, immediate memory is composed of verbal and visual memory and is an indication of one's learning capabilities and alertness. Immediate memories are briefly stored in the parietal lobes.

Working Memory: The ability to retain information. Working memory involves bringing together old and new data. The frontal lobes manage motor control, concentration, problem-solving skills, planning, and retention of knowledge, all functions of working memory.

THE PROBLEM WITH A LACK OF ATTENTION

Feeling less focused doesn't necessarily mean that you are not as smart as you used to be; in fact, it's the people with above-average intelligence who are the first to notice a change in their attention. For example, driving accidents are some of the greatest mortality risks among older adults, and many of them are caused by the following attention errors.

Omissions: a lack of response to a stimulus, such as forgetting to take your foot off the gas pedal.

Commissions: an inappropriate response to a stimulus, such as making a left turn into oncoming traffic.

Reaction Time: an unusually long delay in response to a stimulus, such as driving slowly or hesitating to change lanes.

Variability: an inconsistent response to a stimulus, such as the inability to maintain safe driving speeds on a highway.

CHANGES IN IQ

There are many different ways to define and measure intelligence, because it involves disparate kinds of thinking and uses many parts of the brain. Intelligence combines processing speed, memory, empathy, creativity, and the ability to put all of these together. Some of these abilities are encoded in your DNA, while others are shaped by your individual experiences, learned behavior, and practice. As we get older, the brain loses processing speed. However, in order to preserve or enhance our intelligence, we need to maintain a quick and creative brain.

THE PROMISE OF NEUROPLASTICITY

As scientists, doctors used to hold as a universal truth that we were each born with all the brain cells we were ever going to have or need. While other parts of the body were able to regenerate with age, the cells of the brain would progressively die off as we age. And once they died, they would be gone forever, and there was nothing we could do about it. In this model, the brain was perceived as stagnant, unable to grow, and a decline in brain function with age was inevitable.

Luckily for us, scientists and researchers did not take this "truth" for granted. The latest advances in brain imaging have shown that the brain can grow new cells, just like every other organ in the body. You see new cell growth on your skin every time you get a cut and it heals. The same may hold true for some cells of the brain.

The ability of the brain to change and grow is known as *neuroplas-*

ticity. Plasticity does not refer to being synthetic, or fake. Instead, it refers to being moldable, pliable, and repairable. In this sense, it means that the brain has the capacity to repair itself—to change and grow—through the creation of new neurons and neuronal connections.

Neuroplasticity occurs through a process we call *neurogenesis:* the creation of new neurons. As these brain cells increase and make new connections, you can continue to learn, improve your thinking and your mood, create new memories, and retain cognition well into your old age. In short, we are not predestined to have dementia. You can even train your brain and enhance its abilities, including getting smarter, as you get older. Last, neurogenesis has a positive effect on your overall health, because what is good for the brain is good for the body.

How Do We Know Neuroplasticity Really Exists?

Neurogenesis makes sense theoretically because we can, and do, learn new things all the time. We master new skills, create new relationships, and hone our understanding of both history and current events to make sense of our world. What's innovative is that we now have a scientific pattern that explains new learning as new brain connections.

But for those who need more proof, science has proven neurogenesis exists in relation to our sensory perceptions. In a study financed by the National Institutes of Health (NIH) and published in the *Journal of Neuroscience,* researchers found that when one sense is lost, the corresponding brain region can be recruited for other tasks: those cells don't waste away and die. In deaf people, the part of the brain that is supposed to handle auditory processing is instead recruited to enhance the other senses. Other studies have shown that structural changes in the auditory cortex are noticeable in the brains of deaf children from a very early age. As reported in the *New York Times,* the bottom line is that losing one sense can cause the brain to become rewired, which is neuroplasticity in action.

Reverse an Aging Brain Now: It's Never Too Late to Start

The goal of enhancing brain health is to improve anatomy as well as brain chemistry—both structure and function—by increasing our capability for neurogenesis. At Canyon Ranch, we believe that these kinds of improvements can be made through simple changes in lifestyle. While your genes do play a role in your overall health, many preventive therapies exist that can allow you to keep your brain healthy as you age. This is where epigenetics comes into play—lifestyle changes will transform your health to create a whole new destiny.

The health of the brain is a result of all the positive and negative impacts we've encountered over the course of our lives. The negative aspects include poor health, physical injury like a concussion, and simply following a poor diet. So it's never too early to start to heal the brain, and it's never too late. The truth is, some damage can be repaired if you start to take care of your brain long before you experience the symptoms of cognitive decline. If you don't address these issues, the damage can become permanent. At Canyon Ranch, we prefer to prevent problems with the brain rather than reverse them: it's a lot tougher to reverse damage than to thwart damage.

The goal we are trying to achieve is optimal well-being. In order to reach that, we'll teach you easy ways to be a little more diligent about your lifestyle. We know that people have not lived perfect lives. We can't erase the past, and we certainly don't want to. But at the same time, we're not here to add to your levels of stress. So the first step to better brain health is to take a deep breath and realize that you don't have to be perfect now, either. The rest of this book will teach you what you need to know to become healthier in every way. All we're asking is that you start to take the steps needed to put you on this path. Whatever stage of health you are at right now, you can begin this program.

Over the next thirty days, you'll learn how your current lifestyle may be contributing to poor brain health, or if you are already doing the right things to enhance your cognition. The next chapter discusses physical issues that may be contributing to a decline in brain function. To think of the brain without considering your current physical health is to misunderstand the brain in its entirety. You'll learn that if you take care of your body, you'll have enhanced brain functioning. And when you take care of your brain, you'll have enhanced overall health. The Canyon Ranch philosophy is to address all aspects of your health together—*holistically*—and when you do that, you're going to see results.

Chapter 2

YOUR CURRENT HEALTH AFFECTS YOUR BRAIN

There are many ways that the body's health affects the brain. Some of these relationships are straightforward: a blow to the head resulting from a fall or a sports injury can cause a concussion, which can damage the brain either temporarily or permanently. Others are less obvious but equally dangerous; for example, obesity can be a risk factor for other illnesses, including heart disease and diabetes, both of which can affect your vascular health and ultimately your cognition.

Some of the physical symptoms that you may be experiencing are the result of illness or infection; others can be traced to your genetic code. At Canyon Ranch we don't believe that any illness is related to "normal" aging. However, the most common signs of aging—wrinkles, dry skin, hair loss, hearing loss, visual loss, and arthritic joints—are very real clues that your internal systems are not working as well as they could, and those systems also affect your brain. This chapter will teach you how to determine if your current health is affecting your thinking. Then you'll learn how you can enhance these systems so that you can slow down the body's aging process.

The key is to keep your body healthy so that you will be resilient to disease. When you create a stronger body, you will have a stronger brain. This idea has been repeatedly validated, most recently by two independent studies released in 2013, which linked falling dementia rates in 2013 to areas with the healthiest populations. At the same time, your resilient brain will control the health of the rest of the body. This will not only allow you to retain your good health but will also enable you to keep a high cognitive function well into old age. In one of the two new studies, it was found that healthy people in their nineties were scoring substantially better in 2010 than their cohorts did a decade earlier.

Let's start with the many ways the brain and body are connected. The skull, which is the bone covering of the brain, is part of the skeletal system that provides the framework for the entire body. The spinal cord is attached to the brain stem through a canal in the center of the spine, which houses bundles of nerve fibers. Together with the brain, this forms the *central nervous system*. This system directly connects the brain to the nerves of most parts of the body, creating a network that carries information in the form of electrical signals, which are governed by the various neurotransmitters. These signals control how each of your internal organs works, how quickly and efficiently you metabolize and digest food, and how accurately you respond to stimuli. They also control everything we do, from voluntary actions like walking and talking to the things the body does automatically—like breathing. The central nervous system also transmits sensory information to the brain, which then helps us create emotions, thoughts, and memories.

The brain and the body are also connected through the bloodstream and the lymphatic system. These are pathways that transport fluids, and conditions that affect or travel within the blood and lymph may affect the brain, such as in sepsis (systemic infection) and in some cases, cancer.

Risk Factors That Can Age Your Brain

There are four major risk factors of Alzheimer's disease, which not only affect the end of the spectrum of brain health but can even cause minor dysfunctions you may be currently experiencing. Each factor decreases your brain's ability to process information and maintain a good mood. They are referred to as the Four As of Alzheimer's.

- **Age**
- The **ApoE4** gene
- A diagnosis of **atherosclerosis**
- Inflammation, most commonly seen as **arthritis**

Aging and Hormone Loss

One in eight Americans over age sixty-five is experiencing the signs and symptoms of Alzheimer's disease. For those over seventy-five, the odds of having the disease are one in four, and by the time we are eighty-five, the odds are almost one in two. Some medical professionals would look at these numbers and say that any cognitive decline is simply a factor of aging that's neither curable nor reversible. However, we at Canyon Ranch don't believe this is the case. Instead, we know that identifying poor health and specific risk factors at the earliest stages can help you prepare now for issues that can appear later in life. One of these risk factors that is directly related to aging is declining hormone levels.

Hormones are chemical messengers produced in a variety of glands. Many of these glands are found in the brain, including the pituitary gland, the pineal gland, and the hypothalamus; others are found throughout the body, including the thyroid and parathyroid glands (located at the base of the neck), the thymus (which sits below the sternum), the adrenal glands (found on top of the kidneys), the ovaries (in women), the testes (in men), and the pancreas. The same fluid pathways that connect the brain to the body also allow for the transfer of hormones to help regulate and maintain various body functions. Hormone production occurs as a response to stress and injury, growth and development, absorption of nutrients, energy metabolism, reproduction, birth, and lactation.

When you are young and healthy, you can achieve robust hormone production. But as you age, your hormone levels naturally decline. This is true for both men and women, although women experience a more drastic change during menopause. Scientists and researchers are still trying to decipher the relationship between declining hormone production and cognition. Most of these studies involve the sex hormones: estrogen and progesterone for women and testosterone for men. Many researchers believe that estrogen and testosterone may act as neurotransmitters in the brain and influence cognition and behavior.

Estradiol is a hormone produced in women's ovaries and in smaller amounts in the adrenal cortex, and for men, in the testes. In these areas, estradiol is converted into estrogen. As its production dwindles, menopause occurs, and the brain begins to struggle without it. Imagine that the brain has just lost a chemical it's been dependent on in order to function. Now it has to learn to live without it. During menopause, many women experience changes in their mood, memory, and attention. These women can experience sudden mood swings and "brain fog," an overwhelming feeling of forgetfulness.

However, studies have not shown a clear link between these symptoms and a decline in estrogen, even though we know that estrogen levels drop during menopause. Some researchers believe that estrogen affects the production of the neurotransmitter serotonin, which then impacts mood and memory. Yet we also know that menopausal women don't sleep well, and poor sleep can also affect memory (you'll learn more about this in chapter 5).

We do know that the estrogen levels present in youth help protect women from stroke compared to men of the same age, and this protection is lost within the ten years following menopause. This depletion may indicate that estrogen replacement therapies are a potent element in ongoing neuroplasticity. Unfortunately, they are not without their own drawbacks. Estrogen therapies may be linked to heart disease and cancers, including breast cancer.

For men, the research is equally challenging. Scientific data show that both men and women with Alzheimer's have lower testosterone levels and that low free testosterone may precede Alzheimer's disease. Positive associations have been found between testosterone levels and cognition, memory, executive functions, and spatial performance. It may be that an optimal level of testosterone exists at which some cognitive functions are improved, yet this level has not been identified. Some studies suggest that enhancing testosterone levels to a more physiologically appropriate range makes sense. This suggestion refers to men who have lower testosterone levels than are considered normal for their age, not to enhancing testosterone to levels befitting an earlier stage of life.

Treating Hormone Deficiencies

At Canyon Ranch, we don't believe that just replacing hormones to achieve more youthful levels can cure the symptoms of poor brain health. We strongly believe that certain processes that occur in the body have to be respected, and these include menopause and the gradual loss of hormones in men, known as andropause. We don't believe it is "normal" or even healthy for a seventy-year-old to have the hormone levels of a twenty-year-old.

Philosophically, we believe in an individualized approach to medicine: people have to decide with their own doctor what is the best treatment protocol for their current health and their stage of life. Often, the solution is not necessarily enhancing hormone levels but fixing the reason why these hormone levels might be off. In order to do this, we always start with lifestyle modifications, the same ones that are included in this book. So even before you can start thinking about hormone replacement therapy, you first still need to get your body and your brain clean. Then, to make the best decisions, talk with your doctor and together you can evaluate your current health as well as the risks and benefits of these therapies.

Don't Forget Your Thyroid

The thyroid gland is another big player in a hormone level diagnosis. Hypothyroidism (a decrease in thyroid hormone output) is more commonly found in women. It can cause brain-related symptoms such as fatigue, trouble concentrating, low mood, and poor cognition. In fact, hypothyroidism can present just like dementia. A few simple blood tests can determine if your thyroid is affecting your brain health.

YOUR GENETIC CODE

The human body is composed of trillions of tiny cells, each of which was created from a single cell following conception. In the womb, cells split thousands of times and become specialized based on location—there are cells that make up every body part, from the liver to the brain. Yet each of these specialized cells contains the same *genome,* which is the entire collection of our hereditary information that we received from our parents. This information is encoded as our DNA, and the individual segments carrying this genetic information are called *genes.* Some genes correspond to visible traits, such as eye or hair color. Others are related to biological traits that can't be seen, including blood type and risk for specific diseases, as well as the thousands of basic biochemical processes that compose life.

Each of us is carrying two copies of every gene—one copy from our mother and a second copy from our father. These copies may come in different variations, known as *alleles,* which express different traits. The pairs carry basically the same genetic information; however, there may be slight variations within these genes. If one of these genes is different, it is called a *recessive disease,* and the gene is said to be inherited in a recessive pattern, which is less likely to be manifested as the related disease. However, if only one abnormal gene is needed to produce a disease, it's called a *dominant hereditary disorder.* In this case, if one abnormal gene is inherited from Mom or Dad, the child will likely have the disease. If two parents each have one copy of a recessive disease gene, then each child has a 25 percent (one in four) chance of having the disease. If one parent has two copies of the disease gene and the other has one copy, then each child has a 50 percent (one in two) chance of inheriting the disease.

Some diseases are caused by a *genetic mutation,* which is a permanent change in the DNA sequence. Early-onset Alzheimer's disease—occurring in people between ages thirty and sixty—has been linked to a genetic mutation of the DNA code. Very few people are genetically destined to develop AD. Yet another type of Alzheimer's, known as late-onset (which develops after age sixty), is thought to be caused by a *genetic variant*, a subtle change over time in gene expression that increases or decreases a person's risk for developing a disease or condition.

But even with all our knowledge, it remains very difficult to establish a direct link between specific genes and biological processes or diseases. The truth is that most diseases occur when there is a change in more than one gene or are related to other factors, including outside influences. We now know that genes are strongly influenced by exposure to external factors, including diet, living conditions, exercise, stress, medications, and even environmental toxins. Traumatic events and severe chronic stress can also alter the way genes are turned on or off, and can even affect their inheritability. For example, Norman Cousins, the author of *Anatomy of an Illness*, chronicled how his good humor helped him to win his battle with debilitating chronic disease. He believed, as we at Canyon Ranch do, in the biochemistry of emotions, or as we now call it, the mind-body connection.

As mentioned earlier, the study of these types of influences is known as *epigenetics*—that is, how our environment, daily behavioral choices, and activities can affect the expression of our genes. This discipline has made it scientifically clear that your genetics is not always your destiny. To some extent, we each have the ability to control our own health. So even if you have a genetic predisposition, such as obesity, you may have to work harder than somebody who doesn't carry that same genetic predisposition, but you will still be able to keep yourself slim. And when we are dealing with a disease related to a genetic mutation, it is not a guarantee that you will develop that particular disease.

That said, scientific advances have allowed us to peek into our own futures. When it comes to brain health, we do know that there are specific genes associated with cognitive decline and late-onset Alzheimer's disease, and the most notable is called ApoE4. There are now ten susceptible areas of DNA that may influence your brain health, including ApoE, CR1, CLU, PICALM, BIN1, EPHA1, MS4A, CD33, CD2AP, and ABCA7. If you do have one copy or even both copies of any of these genes, the gene is just one of the increased risk factors for developing Alzheimer's later in life. But having those genes doesn't necessarily mean that you're predestined to get Alzheimer's disease.

Environmental influences—the ways we take care of ourselves—have an impact on genetic expression. The advice in this book, including diet, exercise, supplements, and stress management, not only plays a role in determining your health now but also can influence the way genes are expressed later. Specifically, we do know that the ApoE4 gene is modifiable through basic lifestyle changes. We also know that poor health can lead to DNA damage, which may reduce the expression of other genes involved in learning, memory, and neuronal survival, ultimately affecting our ability to grow new brain cells as we age. Positive epigenetic alterations have also been implicated in managing a wide range of psychological disorders, including anxiety and depression, leading us to believe that the way we live our lives and what we do day in and day out, how we take care of ourselves, how we nurture ourselves, and what kind of relationships we have with other people all play a role in who we ultimately become.

Genetic testing can confirm whether you are carrying the ApoE4 gene. Many people want to know, especially if their father or their mother had late-onset Alzheimer's. Knowing if you're predisposed to that illness may be all the information you need to become more diligent about lifestyle choices that you can make now in order to prevent this gene's expression.

Genetics and Addiction

Another interesting piece of genetic research is the hereditary aspect of addictive behaviors. The behaviors we engage in not only are socially influenced but also can be biologically influenced. What's more, how our brain and body respond to addictive substances—foods, drugs, alcohol, cigarettes—can have a genetic component, which is one of the reasons why bad habits are so hard to break. We strongly believe that willpower is not always the answer to resolving addictions. If you are struggling, seek professional help so that you can get the treatment you deserve.

ATHEROSCLEROSIS AND AN AGING BRAIN

Atherosclerosis, or heart disease, refers to disorders of heart function as well as to the internal network of blood vessels to which the
heart pushes blood. There are many parallels between heart health
and brain health. For people between the ages of fifty and sixty, high
cholesterol and high blood pressure are two of the strongest predictors of memory or cardiovascular trouble down the road. Reducing
high blood pressure has also been shown to reduce the risk of cognitive decline. Even if you have already been diagnosed with memory
problems, control of blood pressure may slow or prevent some of the
progression.

Within every cell of the body is a tiny energy production center
called the *mitochondria*. As oxygen is utilized within the mitochondria
to create energy, extra charged oxygen molecules are released, and
these are called *free radicals*, or *reactive oxygen species* (ROS). We produce free radicals all the time, as a part of normal metabolism. Those
free radicals are controlled by antioxidants that naturally occur in the
body or that we take in through diet. However, if the free radicals are
not neutralized, they create *oxidative stress* and can damage the cell
walls, blood vessel walls, proteins, fats, and even the DNA nucleus of
our cells. Oxidative stress is linked to a host of degenerative diseases
such as heart disease, arthritis, and even Alzheimer's disease. In fact,
most diseases that affect the brain, such as dementia, Parkinson's disease, and Alzheimer's, are usually linked to oxidative stress. However,
there are many ways to minimize free radicals so that you can control
your health, especially through diet and exercise.

Reactive oxygen species influence many biological processes, and
their increased production through oxidative stress plays a role in
hypertension (high blood pressure) and atherosclerosis as it is linked
to plaque formation. Anything you can do to decrease oxidative stress
helps both the heart and the brain. You're improving neuroplasticity
by lowering free radical levels, leading to not just prevention of brain
dysfunction but improvement. The best way to combat free radicals

and oxidative stress is through an antioxidant-rich diet, such as the one outlined in chapter 6.

The second most common cause of dementia is *vascular dementia,* and it doesn't occur in a vacuum: the risk factors for this type of dementia and heart disease are pretty much the same. In 1986, David Snowdon, PhD, began a long-term study of 678 nuns in an attempt to examine the onset of Alzheimer's disease. One significant finding from this famous "Nun Study" was that more than 90 percent of those who suffered one or two mini-strokes on top of the most noticeable signs of Alzheimer's found on autopsy, including amyloid plaques, had trouble with their memory before they died. This may prove that vascular risk factors are some of the biggest predictors of long-term brain health.

The Framingham Heart Study confirms these findings. This ongoing study, which began in 1948, made the first big connection between high levels of cholesterol and heart disease. The researchers behind the study also found that as the number of different heart-related factors increased for particular individuals, so did their risk of cognitive decline. These factors include high blood pressure, diabetes, and obesity. We also know that gaining weight around the middle of the torso is a stronger risk factor for stroke than is an increased total body mass. This is why we firmly believe that staying within a healthy weight, following a nutrient-rich diet, and exercising are good not only for your heart but also for your brain.

Studies have also shown that depression is more common among people with heart disease than those without. That's because depression is linked to increased blood pressure and abnormal heart rhythms, as well as chronically elevated stress hormone levels like cortisol that increase your heart's workload. You need to be mindful of your emotional state: when depression goes up, heart disease goes up.

Signs and Symptoms of Heart Disease

The two most common markers for heart disease are a positive family history (genetics) as well as leading a generally sedentary lifestyle. You also need to be on the lookout for these signs and symptoms:

- A sudden onset of sharp pain in an arm, shoulder, and/or the back or stomach
- Shortness of breath
- Chest pain
- Sudden dizzy spells
- Memory loss
- Anxiety

Controlling Cholesterol Matters

Cholesterol is composed of a waxy, fatlike substance that is actually necessary for your overall health. It is an essential component of every cell that coats and lubricates the body, helping blood to travel in a smooth flow. It is usually produced in the liver, but if the body requires more than the liver can produce, it will create its own cholesterol from the foods we eat. However, if more cholesterol is produced than the body can process and use, it begins to build up in the walls of blood vessels in the form of plaques, much like the amyloid plaques that are a signal of Alzheimer's disease. When this happens, cholesterol turns from a helpful necessity to a harmful substance.

There are two types of cholesterol that affect brain health. "Bad" LDL cholesterol comes directly from the liver and is delivered to the cells of the body and, if overproduced, will line the arterial walls. The "good" HDL cholesterol travels the other way; blood transports this type from the arterial walls to the liver, where it is broken down and removed from the body.

We used to believe that high HDL cholesterol levels were a positive predictor of heart health. Yet we now know that for women who have gone through menopause, HDL loses some of its protective role. One reason might be that HDL molecules exist in a couple of different sizes, just as there are small and big LDL cholesterol particles. In both cases, bigger is better. High levels of HDL cholesterol may help reduce the risk of all cardiovascular disease and, in doing so, may also prevent a decline in memory.

One way to control high LDL cholesterol levels is through diet.

The Brain and Blood Flow

The brain, oddly enough, receives a very constant blood flow. Whether you're just sitting down or working out at the gym, and no matter what your blood pressure is, the brain has a way of maintaining the same circulation. This is referred to as *autoregulation,* and the brain is the only organ in the body that does it. Slight differences in blood flow could drastically damage the brain. That's because the brain has the consistency of toothpaste. It's very soft and very susceptible to changes in the pressure inside the skull. Just adding three ounces of fluid to the brain can cause a hemorrhage, which can kill you.

Foods that are low in fat and high in fiber may be the most effective combination for your heart. Fiber-rich foods act like a scrub brush, cleaning out your colon, controlling blood sugar, pulling fat from your arteries, and raising "good" (HDL) cholesterol levels all at the same time. These foods are discussed in chapter 6.

Vascular Health and Stroke Prevention

Changes in blood flow from the heart to the rest of the body also affect brain health. The vascular system carries oxygen-rich blood away from the heart through blood vessels, arteries, and tiny capillaries into the tissues, and back to the heart through the veins. Blood pressure is a measure of how hard your heart has to work to circulate blood through your body. As the diameter of the blood vessels narrows and the arterial walls stiffen from plaque buildup, you can experience up to a 25 percent increase in blood pressure. This elevation in blood pressure can lead to a heart attack, stroke, aneurysm (a rupture of a blood vessel), or death.

High blood pressure is painless, symptomless, and often unexpected, although there is a strong genetic component. As blood pressure increases, so does cognitive decline. The constricting blood vessels cause a decrease in blood flow and oxygen to the brain, both of which are crucial for its health. A stroke occurs when the blood supply to part of the brain is suddenly interrupted or when a blood vessel in the brain bursts, spilling blood into the spaces surrounding brain cells. Brain cells die when they no longer receive oxygen and nutrients from the blood, or when there is sudden bleeding into or around the brain.

Sometimes a person who notices a precipitous mental decline but didn't experience a full stroke may have suffered from a silent stroke, or even a series of mini-strokes. New research suggests that in some cases, memory loss among the elderly may be due to these so-called silent strokes. Since silent strokes and the volume of the hippocampus appear to be associated with memory loss, stroke prevention may be a means for staving off memory problems as well.

The most important ways to prevent stroke are through lifestyle modifications:

- Lower blood pressure with medications and diet.
- Prevent heart disease through diet and exercise.
- Never smoke cigarettes.

> **Symptoms of a Stroke**
>
> If you see or have one or more of these symptoms, don't wait: call 911 right away!
>
> - Sudden numbness or weakness of face, arm, or leg, especially on one side of the body
> - Sudden confusion or trouble speaking or understanding speech
> - Sudden trouble seeing in one or both eyes
> - Sudden trouble walking, dizziness, or loss of balance or coordination
> - Sudden severe headache

INFLAMMATION AND THE BRAIN

Inflammation is the stress response of the immune system. Its purpose is to protect you from infection, injury, or even stress through a complex process that increases blood flow and brings immune-enhancing cells to areas of the body, or brain, that require healing. White blood cells can be sent to fight off an infection, a nutrient imbalance or deficiency, emotional stress, or lack of sleep; they also respond to a traumatic brain injury, like a concussion. Once the damage is repaired, the inflammation is supposed to subside. Yet even when all your internal systems are working properly, inflammation can actually remain high for several weeks after the infection or insult has been addressed. Many health problems begin when inflammation stays ramped up in one particular area or spreads throughout the body. Heart disease is related to chronic, low-grade inflammation in blood vessels, accelerating the buildup of plaque. Asthma is related to an inflammatory response in bronchial airways, and inflammation may also be associated with the development of many cancers. Any condition that includes –itis in its name involves inflammation—gastritis is stomach inflammation; arthritis is inflammation of the joints. If you have significant arthritis, it may be a signal that there is also inflammation in the brain.

Each organ has its own resident immune system. In the brain, the protective white blood cells are called *microglia*. These cells release chemicals that interfere with intellectual function as a result of an inflammatory reaction, causing cellular death and atrophy. We also know that any inflammation that occurs in the body is bad for the brain. A systemic or chronic infection, such as arthritis, chronic sinus disease, Lyme disease, or strep throat, can affect your thinking. Gum disease or tooth loss can be a hidden cause of smoldering, unremitting inflammation that ultimately affects the brain. When these issues happen, there is a decreased opportunity for neurogenesis and neuroplasticity. Some people believe that Alzheimer's disease can be compared to arthritis of the brain.

Most of us can recognize inflammation as swelling and pain. When you've got bad inflammation, you usually know it. If you've got bursitis, it hurts. If you've got appendicitis, you're sick. We also know that untreated depression is a common source of inflammation, causing pain throughout the body and also in the brain. When people say in those commercials, "Depression hurts," it's true; what's causing the pain is inflammation.

Even very low levels of inflammation can have a negative effect on the brain, and the brain is an organ particularly susceptible to inflammation. This can be seen in the stress response. In a study conducted after the 9/11 attack in New York City, researchers found that people who were the most afraid of a second attack had the most inflammation in their brains. The people who were the least afraid had the least inflammation. This finding is one reason why we know how sensitive the brain is, and how quickly it can recover. If you can reduce anxiety, you can reduce inflammation.

Identifying and Reducing Inflammation

Unfortunately, we can't prevent all types of inflammation: we can't live in a bubble, and we are constantly exposed to illness and infection in our daily lives. It's also impossible to prevent all injuries, even if we are extremely careful. When inflammation happens, our goal is to minimize it. To do so we have to prevent as many infections as we can by staying as healthy as possible. If you have an injury, take care of it so that you get over it quicker. Lower levels of inflammation are easier to control; for example, if your body is trying to fight three or four battles at once and then you get strep throat, you're going to get very sick. However, if you're otherwise healthy and overall inflammation is low, you'll recover much more quickly.

A simple blood test called the C-reactive protein test, or CRP, can generally measure current levels of inflammation in the body, including the brain. Studies suggest that higher chronic levels of inflammation may be associated with a predisposition for a loss of cognitive function later in life. Some of these studies also show that people who have the lowest levels of inflammation have the fewest problems with dementia and memory loss.

Genetics may predispose you to be less or more able to control inflammation, but your lifestyle and environment have a strong influence on the process. Studies show that successfully lowering inflammation has a benefit on the brain as well as the body. In numerous studies, aspirin and other nonsteroidal anti-inflammatory agents have been repeatedly shown to reduce soft tissue and organ inflammation, and this reduction may have a protective effect on the brain. Just blocking inflammation immediately improves brain function.

In order to lower inflammation, we also need to block a chemical, made by the white blood cells, called TNF alpha. This can be accomplished through small changes to your diet. Interestingly, 50 percent of your immune system is found in your gut, and that is why certain foods are very effective at lowering inflammation. Again, a diet high in antioxidants is the first step in boosting your immune system. Liberally using the Indian spice turmeric, adding cayenne pepper to foods, or drinking green tea may block the TNF alpha chemicals. Omega-3 fish oils, found in certain fatty fish and supplements, also have anti-inflammatory properties. You'll learn more about these specific foods in chapter 6.

The most effective type of exercise for lowering inflammation is aerobic, or cardiovascular, exercise. This type of exercise is also thought to be good for the heart because it increases blood flow. Even if you are new to exercise, you can still make a significant difference in your inflammation levels and slow down cell self-destruction.

The Food–Mood Connection

Every time you eat, you're taking in millions of bacteria, any one of which could kill you. A healthy immune system does its job by identifying which harmful bacteria to remove through digestion and elimination—however, when your immune system is compromised, it can't do this job very effectively, and your gut becomes a host to bacteria that can negatively affect your brain's health.

Scientists are now making associations linking the foods we eat—and the way the gut reacts to them—to brain-related conditions such as brain fog, ADHD, depression, and anxiety. For instance, those who suffer from celiac disease—a condition that damages the lining of the small intestine due to an immune response to eating gluten found in wheat, barley, rye, and possibly oats—have a much higher incidence of depression than other populations. Yet when these people remove gluten from their diet, their outlook on life improves. The quieting of the inflammation reverses the impact on the brain.

We also know that as we get older, the body doesn't digest as well, and we don't excrete as well. And because of this, we're creating our own toxic load. We may not be making good food choices. We may be taking medications that affect our digestion, or experiencing more stress with less sleep, all of which changes the composition of our gut. Anything that stresses us affects the health of the good organisms in our bowel. Assuming that as you get older, you're accumulating stressors and bacteria, it stands to reason that if the bacteria are interactive with your immune system, your immune system will become compromised. When your immune system is compromised, inflammation increases.

One of the things that good bacteria do is preserve the lining of the gut, which is only one cell thick. This barrier should be a virtually impenetrable shield between the contents of the gut and the rest of the body. But when the health of the bacteria is compromised, so is the health of this shield. When this happens, we can develop "leaky gut syndrome," whereby molecules that otherwise would not be able to gain entry to the gut can slip through, activating the immune system and causing further inflammation, which may have a negative impact on the brain. At the same time, the balance between good and bad bacteria in our system may change, and other organisms, such as yeast, may overgrow. This syndrome underscores how various organisms live in balance within our body all the time, but when the balance is upset, it can be detrimental to our health.

In order to repair the gut, you need to remove foods you may be sensitive to that provoke inflammation. This can be done by following an elimination diet, and a very effective one is outlined in chapter 4. You may also need to decrease the concentration of bad bacteria and increase the production of good bacteria through probiotic supplementation, which we will discuss in chapter 13. You may also assist in restoring the integrity of the bowel wall by eating foods that contain amino acids, such as yogurt, which can nourish the lining of the gut and helps heal inflammation.

By enhancing the health of your gut you may find that your thinking becomes clearer and that you are more alert after meals. You may also experience an easing of depression and an elevation of mood, and when this happens, your memory might improve as well.

Diabetes: Linking Obesity and Inflammation to Brain Health

Diabetes begins when the body can no longer correctly process the sugars it takes in from carbohydrate-dense foods like white rice, white flour, and potatoes. The body should be able to break down these foods into simple sugars, or glucose, and use this by-product as fuel on the cellular level. The hormone insulin should transport the glucose to the cells. However, when the body does not produce enough insulin, the glucose just sits there, building up in the bloodstream and causing a condition called hyperglycemia, or high blood sugar. This condition sets up a cascade of events that can cause inflammation and plaque deposition within the vascular system, including high blood pressure. At the same time, high blood pressure can contribute to diabetes. And we now know that insulin resistance is also associated with poor performance on memory tests.

Some doctors refer to Alzheimer's disease as type 3 diabetes because it is often found in patients who also have higher levels of insulin and glucose. One study actually performed spinal taps on participants and looked at their memory test results. Researchers were trying to find amyloid plaques as well as increased insulin levels in the spinal fluid. Not surprisingly, they found that the two correlated: the higher the insulin, the higher the levels of amyloid plaque.

OTHER HEALTH ISSUES: BRAIN TRAUMA OR INJURY

Brain trauma has a cumulative effect: each event builds on the next, directly affecting memory and cognition in both the short term and the long term. All the hits we received from our youth to the present day—from falling off a bike to tripping on the stairs—pile up and later affect us, long after the physical bruises have healed.

A concussion can be caused by a direct blow to the head, face, or neck, or elsewhere on the body, with an impulsive force transmitted to the head. It typically results in a rapid loss of neurological function that is short-lived and resolves spontaneously. Concussions do not usually cause visible structural damage to the brain, but that doesn't mean they should be taken lightly. In some cases, concussions can also be associated with physical brain injury such as *subdural hematoma,* an injury where bleeding can occur in the brain or above the brain, below the skull.

The most popular misconception about concussions is that they can be identified only after a loss of consciousness. Any of the following can be a result of a head injury and can contribute to cognitive decline now or later:

- Amnesia
- Behavioral changes (e.g., irritability)
- Depression
- Feeling in a fog
- Headache
- Increased emotionality
- Sleep disturbances or daytime drowsiness
- Slowed reaction times
- Unconsciousness

BRAIN PEAK PERFORMANCE

By understanding the risk factors that can affect the brain, you're taking the first important step to optimizing both your brain's and your body's health. Each of these risk factors actually ages your body faster than your chronological age, so by addressing them, you can begin to slow down the speed of aging. This is very important, because the key to maximizing your ability to maintain and enhance neurogenesis is to keep your brain and your body young, vibrant, and healthy.

The rest of the book is a guide to doing just that. In this chapter, you learned that genetics is not equal to destiny; you can take control of your health by changing your lifestyle. This can be done by addressing the five components of peak performance: medical, nutritional, fitness-related, spiritual, and behavioral. For the best results, we suggest that you take on these facets together, and this is why we created a thirty-day plan that incorporates them all. We've learned over the years that anyone can eat the best foods for brain health, but if people aren't exercising, they can't perform at their peak. The same is true if you exercise but don't take the steps to keep your blood pressure under control. Or you may be physically fit but full of anxiety. All the pieces together produce a positive effect that is much more powerful than any one can accomplish on its own.

However, if you can address only one area at a time, start with the behavioral component, which is featured in the next chapter. By learning how to reduce the stress in your life, you can begin to make space for and achieve better brain health.

Chapter 3

IMPROVE MOOD AND MEMORY
BY DECREASING STRESS

Your emotional state, as well as your current mental health, can affect your memory and attention now and throughout your future. In fact, a brain that is not taxed by depression, stress, or addictive behaviors can continue to grow and develop as we get older.

The connection between retaining memories, neurogenesis, and mood is quite clear. Memories are built and stored in the brain's temporal lobes and the hippocampus, areas that are intimately linked to emotion and mood. The amygdala is where we store powerful emotions such as disgust and fright and is connected to memory areas where we interpret faces and emotional expression. Another area, called the *anterior cingulate cortex,* is where we analyze an incoming stimulus for emotional content as well as regulate blood pressure and heart rate. This is the area responsible for mapping out past memories and making predictions based on them. By utilizing these neighboring regions at the same time, the brain is constantly connecting memory, mood, and emotions as it cross-references them so we can make new decisions. What's more, this process allows us to access and store memories based on sensory experiences (smell, touch, sight, sound, and taste), as well as their emotional content; that is why we have happy memories as well as sad ones, and everything in between.

Post-traumatic stress disorder (PTSD) is one of the clearest ways to demonstrate the memory/emotion/mood connection. PTSD is defined as a type of anxiety disorder that occurs after one has seen or experienced a traumatic event that involved the threat of injury or death. After combat, soldiers may suffer from PTSD, but it can also affect anyone who has survived physical or emotional abuse. During the traumatic event, the brain's survival mechanism instantly turns on and releases the chemicals adrenaline and noradrenaline. Adrenaline mediates the fight-or-flight response and gives you the energy to get out of harm's way. Noradrenaline also has a stimulating effect that fosters alertness, and plays an important role in long-term memory and learning. An excess of noradrenaline can fuel fear and anxiety and, at the same time, aids in intense memory consolidation. These chemicals assist the brain in connecting the memory of the traumatic event with your emotional state during that event, so when the memory is recalled later, so are the corresponding emotions. Sufferers report that they feel as if they are reliving the event over and over in their mind, as if it were still happening.

Many also report that during a traumatic event they experience the sensation that time slows down, even though they know this isn't possible. What is really happening is that changes in your memory density are occurring. Again, the brain chemical noradrenaline drives the memory system to store more memories than usual. Because in that instant you are capturing many more memories than you are used to, and they are firmly implanted in your brain because of the emotional connection, you notice every detail of the event, so that it seems as if time were slowing down.

STRESS AND ANXIETY AFFECT MEMORY

While PTSD is on the far end of the anxiety spectrum, everyday stresses can not only create anxiety but affect your ability to remember and prematurely age your brain. This is because we become distracted by our anxieties. If you are constantly trying to juggle six balls at once, it's really hard to keep your focus on all six, especially if you are worried about keeping them in the air. The same is true when people are under stress. When you are overloaded with work or family issues, or when you are anxious about something, you can become distracted and forgetful. Or you can't focus as well, and you begin to make errors in judgment. This doesn't mean that you're developing dementia; it just means that you may have too much on your plate.

We know that stress negatively affects the brain. At Canyon Ranch we see stressed-out people who are operating in survival mode. They feel frenetic and exhausted. They can't think clearly because they don't have the resources; the brain's response to stress is to shut down everything except those systems that are going to keep you alive.

Stress can be acute—short term—or chronic. Memory issues connected to short-term stresses can easily correct themselves once the stress ends. For example, if you are working on a tight deadline, you may not think about the rest of the world—or even the rest of the details in your life—until you've met your goal. Once you have, your attention and memory return.

However, if you're under prolonged, chronic stress, your brain begins to compensate with another survival mechanism. During periods of chronic stress, the neurotransmitters, or brain chemicals, that are vital for healthy cognitive function become depleted. These include the chemicals that power your brain, such as dopamine, epinephrine, and acetylcholine, the neurotransmitter that's most responsible for attention and memory. To make up for the loss of brainpower, the pituitary gland inside the brain signals the adrenal gland, located above the kidneys, to release a replacement hormone known as cortisol. This hormone is produced in greater quantities when we are stressed, and provides the energy our brain needs to continue to function. The good news is that our brains are well-suited to manage small doses of cortisol; however, elevated levels of cortisol overstimulate the brain, and this overstimulation eventually depletes you emotionally, physically, and intellectually. Worse, too much cortisol can change the physical structure of the brain, causing the hippocampus to shrink. This is a problem because the hippocampus is the part of the brain most important for short-term memory. In order to maintain your ability to create and store memories, it's vitally important to manage your stress and cortisol levels.

Cortisol causes dendrites to retract. You may remember that the dendrites are the single-eyed projections that allow neurons to communicate quickly with other brain cells. When you retract those dendrites, retrieving stored information becomes harder. High levels of cortisol also cause a certain degree of cell death because when you're chronically stimulated, you're releasing a large amount of the amino acid glutamine. Glutamine causes the cells to open up and allow in a rush of calcium, which helps the chemical message move from one cell to the next. But if a cell gets too much calcium, it may die. This is why the creation of new neuronal connections takes place to a lesser extent when you are under stress.

Cortisol also affects the amygdala, which is the part of the brain that ties an emotion to an experience or memory. High cortisol levels actually cause the amygdala to grow up to an additional inch in size, making these connections even more powerful and creating a higher degree of anxiety over nerve-racking experiences.

Other hormonal changes can also cause stress and anxiety—for example, women going through menopause can become stressed because of the changes they are experiencing, and the stress then increases cortisol production. At the same time, the hormones estrogen and progesterone are decreasing. In terms of brain health, progesterone is critical, because it is a very soothing and calming hormone. Without it, you will lose that beneficial armor of calmness.

DEPRESSION

Our personalities and worldviews absolutely influence the ways our brains age. People who are more curious about life and who handle stress well are going to be able to maintain better brain health as compared with those who are not interested in learning new things, who are pessimistic and cynical and get angry all the time, and who are loaded with stress. We know this is true because depression is also linked to the overproduction of cortisol. In one 2003 study published in the *American Journal of Psychiatry,* the volume of the hippocampus was less in people who had depression than in people of the same age and the same health who didn't have depression. However, when the depression was treated, whether with medications or psychotherapy, researchers actually saw a rebound in terms of the hippocampal volume, suggesting there is some degree of reversibility. The findings also showed that antidepressants, when used appropriately, may have a neuroprotective effect.

We also know that stressful events promote neurochemical changes that may be involved in the provocation of depression. What's more, people who are profoundly depressed act as if they have dementia. When we are depressed, there's an overactivation of certain brain regions, such as the ones responsible for worrying, and an underactivation of others, such as the hippocampus and certain parts of the prefrontal cortex, which can cause the symptoms of dementia. People with low mood may find it hard to think, and the deeper a person is in depression, the harder it is to think clearly. This condition then affects memory, attention, and judgment. If people suffer from obsessive-compulsive behavior or thoughts, they may fixate on one topic and not pay attention to the rest of what is going on around them. Or they start having intrusive negative thoughts.

It's difficult to determine if depression causes the symptoms of dementia, or if dementia causes depression, in older adults. Some become depressed when they lose brain function, or when they realize that their lives are more limited. Neurologists and psychologists agree that enhancing mood is a good initial step, regardless of which condition came first. By treating the depression, they find that cognitive function can get better.

ADDICTION

The brain creates habits and addictions in a process that involves a three-step activity loop called the *dopamine reward system,* which releases the brain chemical dopamine in anticipation of exposure to pleasure. First, there is a cue or trigger that excites your brain. Then there is the routine, which can be a physical, mental, or emotional event. Finally, there is a reward, which helps your brain solidify the event as worth remembering for the future. Over time, this loop becomes more and more automatic, and a habit emerges. The habit can be something as simple as kissing your spouse or partner good night. But when the cue and reward become neurologically intertwined, a sense of craving emerges, and suddenly, habits become addictions. The release of dopamine creates a surge of excitement, or a "rush" in anticipation of the reward. Alcohol, cocaine, heroin, marijuana, nicotine, amphetamines, Ecstasy, OxyContin, and glucose (from overconsumption of simple carbohydrates) all cause a release of dopamine, as do addictive behaviors like gambling, shopping, or even sex.

Habits can be ignored, changed, or replaced. But unless you deliberately replace a habit with new cues and rewards, the old pattern will return; this is why addictive substances and behaviors are linked to memory. Studies performed at the National Institutes of Health show that just by thinking about a vice, the brain releases a small amount of dopamine and links it to the memory and the "good feeling" emotion. Once you've experienced a good "rush," your memory craves the experience again. So not only do you become addicted to the substance, you become addicted to the dopamine release.

However, when we develop addictive behaviors, they actually make us less happy. Frequent exposure to addictive behaviors and substances decreases the number of dopamine receptors in the brain. With fewer receptors, lower levels of dopamine are activated, leaving more intense cravings and increased stress. Over time, it takes a larger exposure of whatever you are addicted to in order to reach the level of reward. The catch is that the brain can't keep up with demand. Instead, it strives to reach homeostasis, or balance, so that each time you are exposed to the addictive substance or behavior, the brain releases less dopamine, not more. When this happens, the euphoric feeling doesn't come back at all. Yet many people will still continue to drink or smoke in the hope that it will return.

What's more, many addictive substances directly cause cognitive failures. Alcoholics are known to experience blackouts, which are memory gaps that occur even when they are conscious. Both illegal street drugs and prescription pain medications can tamper with memory, cloud judgment, limit attention, and increase forgetfulness. The long-term damage of drug and alcohol addiction is related to cognitive decline as it both kills off brain cells and disrupts brain chemical production, which is directly linked to dementia. Surprisingly, it doesn't take much to create damage: in a 2011 study from Northumbria University, people who smoked cigarettes only on weekends caused as much damage to their memory as those who smoked on a daily basis.

Some people will try to self-medicate their low mood or anxiety with alcohol, drugs, or food. Many come home from a hard day of work and pour themselves a few drinks in order to release the tension of the day. Unfortunately, the strategy they've chosen may offer temporary relief, but can cause bigger health problems down the road, such as obesity, liver disease, and cognitive decline. Addiction is serious, and it can require professional help. When you develop addictive behaviors, you have to identify them so you can stop them. If you believe you have an addiction, talk to your doctor to find the right programs that address your particular health issues.

LETTING GO OF STRESS

Successful aging and maintaining a healthy, active brain depend on avoiding stress, anxiety, depression, and addiction. Medications may help, and you should talk to your doctor about your specific mental health issues in order to craft a plan to treat these conditions.

You can also learn to reduce stress and anxiety by changing your behavior. This in turn can help you become stronger, more resilient, and hopefully, even happier. Resilience is an important part of your long-term brain health. We all have to deal with adversity in life; however, if we look at the brains of happy, resilient people, we can see that they function differently from those of people who are chronically unhappy or stressed. Happy people display more activity in the left prefrontal cortex, where you rationalize and make decisions. In contrast, during times of anxiety, blood flow activity shifts away from the prefrontal cortex and toward the middle of your brain, where adrenaline is released, forcing your thoughts to go from rationalization to reaction. This is why it is so hard to stop a panic attack once it has begun, and why staying calm in the face of adversity is key to maintaining a healthy, thinking brain.

The following strategies are ways Canyon Ranch works with our guests to reduce and relieve stress. You can explore each or all of them, or come up with your own. Any strategy that allows you to calm yourself, and that you can call upon whenever you are feeling stressed or anxious, will work. Many of them can help promote neurogenesis on their own, making them additionally beneficial.

We can't always minimize stress, but we can modify how we respond to it and how we allow it to affect us. So if you are having a stressful day or you're in a very stressful situation, having these techniques and tools in your pocket allows you to pull yourself out of a potentially bad situation and then make a change in a meaningful way. It's amazing how different you can feel after just a few minutes of calm.

Get Rid of the Word Stress

The bestselling author Dr. Wayne Dyer believes there isn't any one thing that is "stress." It's really a made-up word that encompasses everything we consider to cause a negative emotion. He writes that many people confuse frustration, impatience, rage, depression, isolation, panic, and terror with stress. However, these are all emotional responses that we can and should deal with in order to achieve happiness. We at Canyon Ranch view stress as the difference between where you are and where you actually want to be.

When people come to Canyon Ranch, one of the first things we teach them is to take the word *stress* out of their vocabulary and begin to name whatever it is that they are feeling. If you can get rid of the word *stress* and instead focus on naming the emotion or physical pain that underlies it, you will help yourself release the anxiety that accompanies it. We can't always solve our problems immediately, but identifying them does help.

Instead of saying, "I'm totally stressed out," it is more reasonable to say any of the following that accurately identifies your current state: "I'm feeling sick in my gut." "I'm feeling tight in my throat." "I feel as if I'm going to cry." "I'm hurt because of this situation at home." "I'm overburdened with work."

Reframing

In the past ten years, researchers have discovered that experiences can change the way neurons fire in our brains. If traumatic experiences can change our brains, as in PTSD, many mental health professionals are suggesting that positive relationships can restore and possibly enhance our brain health. This type of therapy is referred to as positive psychology, or interpersonal neurobiology (IPNB). Clinicians report that new positive emotional relationships, as well as reframing old ideas or habits, will lead to substantial changes in your mood and behaviors. For example, we know that depression often stems from false thinking and negative self-talk; we convince ourselves of things that aren't necessarily true. However, if you can focus on the things that make a difference to your personal happiness, instead of dwelling on the things that make you unhappy, you will become more resilient in the face of adversity, and greater resilience in turn will allow you to better handle stressful situations. One way to do this is to link experience to memory and try to remember things positively. This makes a huge difference in how you feel and how you will think about your memories.

When you're stressed about work and begin to think, "I hate my job, I hate my job, I hate my job," you can reframe that thought and say to yourself, "I still hate my job but my chair is comfortable. I'm one of the lucky people who have a job. I am working at this job so that my kids can eat."

Reframing allows you to feel centered so that you can live in the moment, and by doing so, you are more likely to feel better about yourself. You're not living in fear of everybody. You're not suspicious. You trust people. When we resist what's actually happening in our lives, we create a much more stressful response. Instead, you have to learn how to accept what's actually happening and choose to be optimistic, focusing on the lessons and the opportunities for growth instead of the problem.

Spend Time with Friends

People who are more socially engaged tend to stay more cognitively healthy. There are two reasons why this may be true. The first is that they're getting more stimulation. They are people who are having conversations, who are thinking on their feet—and all of that stimulates the brain. Second, as long as the social connections are emotionally satisfying, then they enhance mood and decrease stress. Studies have also shown that people who are profoundly lonely produce excess cortisol.

While we all try to choose our friends wisely, in terms of brain health, the most important aspect of picking friends is that you choose to spend time with emotionally healthy people. The brain has a unique mirroring ability: it quite literally takes an imprint of the habits of those you spend time with and mirrors back their behaviors through your own actions. It's almost as if your brain is trying on your friends so that you can feel what it might be like to be them. We end up mimicking each other's body postures, breathing patterns, and worldviews. So surround yourself with positive, calm, resilient people, and you will learn to become one.

Go Out of Your Way to Relax

Make time to actively get rid of the stress and anxiety you create, and you'll lower cortisol levels. It's well documented that you can improve mood through physical activity, and you'll learn more about that in chapter 7. There is also evidence that breath work, which we will discuss in chapter 8, can relax the mind. Yet there are other physical ways to relieve stress. One of the most popular at Canyon Ranch is through massage. In a 2010 overview published in the *Journal of Clinical Psychiatry*, seventeen individual studies showed that massage therapy is significantly associated with alleviating depressive symptoms, although we are still not sure how it actually helps. The science and practice of massage therapy have evolved significantly over the years, and now more than twenty different types of massage therapies are offered at Canyon Ranch.

Neurofeedback is another technique that can relax the brain so you can focus. A neurofeedback session feels like a comforting experience in a futuristic setting. Sensors are placed on your head in key spots to read the speed of brain waves. The ratio of speed and amplitude from front to back and side to side should ideally be in balance, and this technology allows you to practice techniques to achieve that. With the sensors in place, you are shown a soothing image, such as a sailboat, accompanied by sound. Therapists can see how your brain waves react to these images, and from there, you can learn how to control brain energy to achieve balance and improve attention and focus.

Go Outside

Another effective way for you to ease the stress response is by literally changing your view. Just sitting quietly outside for a few minutes can help. Nature is easy on the eyes and easy on the ears, and by linking yourself to its calmness, you can lower your anxiety. Take the time to notice what the shadows look like, what the green of the grass looks like, or the different smells of the seasons. Nature is always changing, and by focusing your attention outward, outside yourself and into the world, you make space to engage other parts of the brain in new and profound ways that can help ease the burden of whatever it is you left behind. This is why we strongly believe that just being in nature is probably one of the most powerful medicines we have. Whether you listen to the sound of the ocean or a quiet rain, pulling yourself out of your hectic life—even for a few minutes—can help reset your mood and create a sense of release.

Get Creative

Creativity not only reduces stress and anxiety, it generates neuroplasticity and helps to keep the brain robust. It can facilitate new neuronal connections because whenever you do something creative, you're putting old information together in new and different ways. This way of thinking has been frequently attributed to the wisdom of aging, where we create new paradigms from information that is available. That's why the aging brain and the creative brain are very similar ideas.

One of the marvelous things about enhancing creativity is that we don't have to be talented in order to enjoy it. It's the process, not the outcome, that enhances our brain and decreases stress. In fact, creativity is not about crafting great works of art. Once you internalize the idea of letting go of perfection, you can find the process satisfying. Embracing the learning curve allows you to move toward excellence, whereas the perfection model is very rigid, tight, and constraining.

What's more, it doesn't matter if you're motivated to create a wonderful meal or a piece of music or just to play the guitar or to find a new way of doing something different in your life. Being creative can include writing a poem, working with clay, baking, drawing, beading, painting, or simply looking at the world differently. All that is important is finding a good fit that combines your interests with your imagination.

One of the most creative outlets that almost anyone can participate in is dance. Most of us have warm memories of dancing with people we love because dance is a single-focus, sensory experience that imprints a deep memory, so that you have a positive connection to it. Dance is so effective because you have to be completely present and in the moment in order to enjoy it. And it's a perfect brain exercise because it involves processing sight, sound, rhythm, focus, balance, memory, self-control, interpersonal feedback, and creative experimentation. At Canyon Ranch we offer exercise dance classes because they increase not only cardiovascular health but also mood. What's more, when people return to the ranch and take the same classes again, we know they have created a positive memory. And while these classes work for our guests here, twenty minutes of turning on your favorite high-tempo music and dancing around your living room when nobody is watching will have the same positive effect, right in your own home.

Listen to Music

Music has the ability to alter mood dramatically and positively, so it only makes sense that it can have an impact on your brain. Music can calm the brain and allow it to succumb to sleep. Like dance, music offers a sensory experience that gives you a reprieve from your overengaged mind. However, you have to choose music that truly resonates with you in order for it to alter your mood.

Keep a Journal

Writing has a huge impact on emotional states. One exercise that channels writing positively is creating a gratitude journal as a measurable way to quantify happiness. Gratitude is a powerful emotion that can shift your entire attitude toward life and can be mood enhancing. Martin Seligman, PhD, who is one of the pioneers in positive psychology, suggests that people can learn to recognize happiness by counting their blessings. Participants in his research were asked to write down five things they should be grateful for each day for five days. The outcome for the participants was that they felt as if they were "inoculated against depression" for up to six months. You can participate in the exercise by drawing two columns on a piece of paper: one headed "Blessings," and the other marked "Reason." At the end of each day for the next week or so, write down three things that happened that you feel grateful for in the Blessings column. These don't have to be big things; they can be as simple as "I got to work on time" or as big as "My daughter had a healthy baby boy." In the Reason column, write down why you think the good thing happened. For example, if you wrote, "I got to work on time," it could be because "My kids cooperated" or perhaps "I woke up early and got out of bed." Another journaling activity is to write testimonials to people who have made a difference in your life. This is another form of the "count your blessings" exercise, where you show how thankful you are for the people in your life.

Other people feel comfortable releasing stress effectively by writing about it. You don't have to share these entries with anyone else, although many people find that the act of sharing their writing is what releases the stress, because they feel it removes the negative energy.

Try Something New

Novelty relates to the mental curiosity that is very much a part of the human condition and that we need in terms of creating brain growth. We all need to foster a little mental flexibility so we do not get stuck in a rut of doing things only one way. We can easily become so habituated and patterned into our life that we don't even think about going to the dairy section first if we always go to the vegetable section first. Or if we always go to this gas station rather than that gas station, we'll always take the same route home. Trying new things allows us to create a different kind of mental stimulation and can help us break the cycle of stress that accompanies repetition. It's not necessary just to do the things you are good at; it's also critical to try new things in order to cultivate mental flexibility.

Find the Love

Love and stress are probably at opposite ends of a spectrum: the feeling of being loved and receiving love is the opposite of stress. Just as stress increases the production of cortisol, we know that being in the presence of love creates a more positive atmosphere within the brain that can trigger the release of the hormone oxytocin, the love hormone. Oxytocin is released when you feel safe and secure, when you are transmitting and receiving tenderness through eye gaze or touch, and during sex. It provides a wash of calmness over the brain and the body.

Loving relationships alter the brain the most significantly. A happy marriage relieves stress and makes you feel more resilient in the face of adversity. Outside of a loving relationship, you can pinpoint the things in life that make you happy. And if you can do one of those things every day, it can unquestionably improve mood. It will help you to maintain your cognitive ability, and it will be good for your brain. And people who are good at being happy handle stress better.

Ask for Help

Because we're a very independent culture, we have a collective tendency to think that we must solve problems or deal with crises alone. Yet the brain is constantly searching for a companion. Intrinsically, we need other people just as much as we need to understand a source that's larger than us. And just as you strive for companionship, it is often the best medicine to ask for help when you need it. This is especially true if you find yourself in a situation that makes you anxious or stressed. Medical professionals and therapists, as well as family and friends, can lend a hand in lightening your burden or providing assistance so that you can figure out the best course of action.

Once you can get a better handle on releasing stress and anxiety, you can begin to work on another pillar of peak performance. In the next chapter, you'll see how both the medical and the nutritional aspects of optimizing health come together in order to detoxify the brain and the body.

Chapter 4

A TOXIC ENVIRONMENT
AFFECTS YOUR THINKING

Doctors and researchers have long recognized that a toxic environment can affect our overall health. Children growing up in cities with high levels of air pollution tend to have more asthma, and certain chemical exposures, such as tobacco smoke, are linked to cancer. In addition, toxic foods—including some processed foods as well as those high in sugar—are directly linked to chronic diseases like obesity, diabetes, and more. But the relationship between toxins and brain function has been more difficult to prove, although we at Canyon Ranch strongly believe that their effects can be just as detrimental.

One of the main problems in identifying how toxins affect brain health is that each of us handles every type of exposure differently. In just the same way that two people can follow an identical eating program and one will lose weight and the other will gain, we suspect that some people are simply more susceptible to toxins, and that others are more resilient.

The toll toxins take on our health also depends on the amount of toxins we have accumulated over the years. We call this the *body burden*. Some chemicals stay with us for only a short time before we effortlessly remove them through the intestines, kidneys, or lungs or through the skin as sweat. However, before they are eliminated, the molecules of many fat-soluble toxins have to undergo a transformation that makes them less harmful and water soluble, in a process called *detoxification.* Most detoxification happens in the liver.

Continuous or repeated exposure to these chemicals makes it harder for the body to detoxify, simply because they can overwhelm the liver's capacity to do its job. Other toxins remain in our blood and brain tissue forever because the body is just not capable of removing them. Eating an occasional meal of tuna or swordfish—both of which may be high in the element mercury—will not be likely to have any effect on your cognition; however, if you eat these fish daily and your body can't remove the mercury efficiently, then it is more likely that the mercury will build up in your system and negatively affect your health.

The same toxins can cause more significant damage to children and developing fetuses. Even the amount of toxins a woman accumulates in her body prior to becoming pregnant will have an impact on her baby. We call this a *transgenerational effect,* and for many toxins it is worse than the impact the same toxin would have on the mother. While we do not have a clear explanation of why so many of our children suffer from a host of mental health issues, ranging from depression to attention deficit hyperactivity disorder (ADHD) to autism, we must be open to the possibility that our increasingly toxic environment may be responsible to some extent.

Sometimes, it's not one particular toxin but a combination of various toxins that may lead to brain problems and other health concerns. Scientists at the Environmental Protection Agency (EPA) estimate that we are carrying more than seven hundred contaminants inside our bodies at any given time, regardless of whether we live in a rural area, a large city, or near an industrialized zone. Their negative effect is not just cumulative but exponential, as some toxins can actually make others even more potent. This reaction is called *synergistic toxicity.*

Some of us are just naturally better than others at detoxifying. Whether you are a good or a bad detoxifier is influenced by your genetics, your lifestyle (diet, exercise, amount of stress), and your current health status. You may be an excellent detoxifier, and though you are exposed to the same toxins as your neighbor, you will be completely fine and healthy and will live to be a hundred. Meanwhile, your neighbor, who is less adept at detoxification, may become sick instantly or experience symptoms later.

The way you respond to stimuli in your everyday life can help you estimate how well your body is eliminating toxins—for example, if one cup of coffee makes you jittery, you may be a poor detoxifier, because the caffeine is not leaving your system efficiently. Or if you take over-the-counter medications that are categorized as stimulants, like some decongestants, and your heart races after taking even the smallest of doses, you may be a poor detoxifier. If you enter a freshly painted room and suddenly get a headache, you may be a poor detoxifier. These sensitivities are also signs that your brain may be affected by your environment.

Another problem with establishing a clear relationship between toxins and poor brain health is that some of the most dangerous chemicals do not immediately cause symptoms. In fact, there can be as much as several decades between an exposure and the diagnosis of its related disease. Worse, many of these most dangerous toxins are persistent in the environment: they stay there forever. One study conducted by the Environmental Working Group showed that when people were tested to determine their "toxome," or the identity of the various toxins in their blood, they presented an average of two hundred toxins, many of which were chemicals like polychlorinated biphenyls (PCBs) that have been banned for more than thirty years.

New studies are being released every year that confirm our suspicions that toxins can affect our memory, attention, and mood. One important study released in 2012 links air pollution more directly to declining memory and attention. In the Nurses' Health Study cognitive cohort, researchers followed older women for more than a decade and found that higher levels of long-term exposure to typical air pollution were associated with significantly faster cognitive decline in measures of memory and attention span. The highest exposures had the same effect on the brain as if it had aged prematurely by as much as two years. While this doesn't sound like much, our goal is to keep you living younger longer, not aging faster.

How Toxins Affect the Brain

The most common causes of oxidative stress are overeating, a lack of antioxidants in the diet, and exposure to environmental toxins. Compared with other tissues in the body, the brain may be the most sensitive to the effect of toxins, particularly those that are fat soluble, as the brain is mostly made of fat. If you want to keep your brain healthy, you must limit exposure to toxins so that you can minimize your body burden, and thus also minimize your levels of oxidative stress.

First, let's identify which toxins are affecting your brain health, so that you know where they are and how to avoid them. Then you'll learn methods to enhance your body's detoxifying abilities so that you can eliminate the toxins you have already been exposed to. The more we understand how we truly live in a toxic world, the better able we will be to minimize the impact the environment has on our health. The following section lists many of the most likely culprits.

Plasticizers

Phthalates and bisphenol A (BPA) are two varieties of plasticizers, industrial chemicals that are used in the manufacturing of plastic products. According to the Environmental Working Group, BPA is used in the production of thousands of products made of hard, clear polycarbonate plastics and tough epoxy resins, including safety equipment, eyeglasses, computer and cell phone casings, water and beverage bottles, the lining of aluminum cans, and certain paints. BPA-based plastics break down easily, particularly when heated or washed with strong detergent. These chemicals can leach into food that is heated or stored in plastic wrap or plastic containers. They can also seep into the environment when these plastics deteriorate. Plastic shopping bags are a huge problem because over time and with exposure to the sun they will break down and contaminate both soil and waterways. If you ever drank water from a plastic bottle that was sitting in the sun, that funny taste was the phthalates that bled into your water from the bottle.

One of the reasons plasticizers are harmful is that they are categorized as *endocrine disrupters*: substances that interfere with the synthesis, secretion, transport, binding, or elimination of natural hormones in the body. One example would be xenoestrogens, chemicals whose molecular structure resembles estrogen, a hormone that men and women naturally create. We have thousands of estrogen receptors throughout the body and the brain. When we are exposed to a xenoestrogen, it interferes with the normal function of these receptors, by either stimulating them excessively or blocking them altogether. In breast tissue, a xenoestrogen can stimulate breast cancer growth; in the uterus, it might lead to fibroids or uterine cancer; in men, it can cause infertility or prostate enlargement. In our brains, these chemicals can lead to changes in behavior. Without the right production of estrogen, our thinking can be negatively affected in much the same way that menopausal women experience brain fog or memory loss. The resulting damage seems to be cumulative: if we were overexposed to xenoestrogens during childhood, they may affect our thinking later in life.

What's more, we know that naturally produced estrogen, as well as other hormones, is integral to the processes of neurogenesis. To keep your brain healthy, you want to stimulate the growth of new brain cells, not diminish it.

> **Choose the Safest Plastics**
>
> The triangular "recyclable" labels on plastic bottles and containers are the best way to know which are the safest to use. At Canyon Ranch, we try to limit plastics whenever possible. But when we do use them, we choose products that are labeled 1, 2, 4, or 5. We suggest you try to avoid plastic wraps, Styrofoam cups or containers, and other products labeled with numbers 3, 6, and 7.

Pesticides, Herbicides, and Fungicides

The main aim of these chemicals is to kill things that bother us, and their targets range from small animals and insects to weeds and mold. Unfortunately, they are all too effective, and their residue finds its way into our food supply. Typically, these chemicals are sprayed into the air, where they can remain on the plants we eat or the feed that cows, chickens, and pigs consume. In the water they are ingested by algae, which are in turn eaten by fish.

Once they enter our food supply, these chemicals then get stored in our fatty tissue, including the brain, where they can damage the brain's nerve cells, causing a disruption in the connection between the synapses and affecting the neurotransmitters. When one particular neurotransmitter called dopamine gets disrupted, your memory retrieval time slows down, and you lose the ability to think quickly. This results in a range of brain health issues, from attention loss to the inability to initiate movement.

Some pesticides known as *organochlorines* (like DDT) and *organophosphates* have been linked to hyperactivity, IQ deficits, memory impairments, developmental delays, and behavioral disorders. Although DDT was banned in the United States in 1972, it is still persistent in our environment because other countries continue to use it. According to the Environmental Protection Agency, DDT can remain in the environment for as many as fifteen years and is still found in fish caught in the Great Lakes region of the United States.

Even seemingly benign products can possibly affect your body burden and brain health. We don't think of antibacterial soaps, chlorine, and fluoride as pesticides, but in the broadest sense, that is exactly what they are. These chemicals serve a useful purpose by eliminating harmful microbes; however, there is some evidence that in some forms they can be toxic to humans over time. So while we don't advocate that you stop swimming or brushing your teeth, think about your daily exposure and consider if they can be negatively affecting your health.

Heavy Metals

Heavy metals are physically dense and sometimes cancer-causing natural elements that include lead, cadmium, arsenic, chromium, and mercury. They are also known to be toxic to the brain and are implicated in brain health issues ranging from headaches to fatigue to oxidative stress and neurodegeneration. Both cadmium and lead have been linked to learning disabilities and decreased IQ. Lead exposure can also cause impulsivity and violent behavior. Mercury has been linked to attention deficit, learning disabilities, and memory impairment as well as motor dysfunction.

Many studies support the correlation between a large, single exposure to any of the heavy metals and damage to the brain. However, continued exposures over many decades to even minute quantities may also have a cumulative effect. Worse, the exposure to several different heavy metals in combination can affect our health, even in minuscule doses. In a 1978 study, one hundred mice were given doses of mercury that killed only one of them. Then the remaining mice were given a small dose of lead, which again killed only one of them. Finally, the remaining mice were given a small dosage of lead and mercury together, which resulted in the death of 100 percent of them.

Recurrent exposure to lead can affect your thinking and cognition. Any house built before 1978 may still contain lead paint and lead plumbing, exposing you daily to particles in the air or in your tap water. Small quantities of lead can also be found in places you would never suspect, including personal cosmetics, toys, and the soil around your home.

Mercury is present in some dental fillings, lightbulbs, and as mentioned, large fatty fish. Dental amalgam is the largest contributor of neurotoxic mercury exposure and affects more than 120 million Americans. Mercury has been the most studied and most closely linked heavy metal that affects brain health, yet the symptoms cover a wide range of complaints that can also be attributed to other health concerns. If you are experiencing any of the following symptoms without relief and are eating lots of fatty fish or believe that you have silver-colored dental fillings containing mercury, see chapter 9 for information on getting tested for mercury poisoning:

- Depression
- Difficulty concentrating

- Disturbances of taste or smell
- Excitability
- Fatigue
- Fearfulness
- Indecisiveness
- Insomnia
- Irritability
- Melancholy
- Memory changes
- Restlessness
- Shyness
- Speech defects

> **Helpful Detox Apps**
>
> One way to minimize mercury exposure is to know what seafood is safe to eat, and in what quantities. The Monterey Bay Aquarium updates such information on a regular basis on its website. You can even download its free Seafood Watch application onto your phone. Go to www.monterey bayaquarium.org/cr/seafoodwatch. aspx for more information.

Make Sure Your Home Is Healthy

Indoor air can also be hazardous to the brain. Residual chemicals from heating and cooling systems, tobacco and cigarette smoke, asbestos, mold, household cleaners, personal care products, and air fresheners can combine to create a toxic indoor environment. Even small bottles of nail polish, deodorants, and other "fragrance" products contain dangerous phthalates. None of these sources alone is strong enough to affect our thinking; however, in combination they have more potency.

Electromagnetic pollution comes from wireless devices and a variety of electric sources, such as power lines, computers, plasma TVs, dimmer switches, energy-efficient lighting, cordless phones, smartphones, wireless routers, and cell phone/broadcast antennas. This type of pollution is somewhat controversial, and studies have not yet been conclusive. However, many people who believe they are affected by electromagnetic frequencies complain of symptoms that include fatigue, headaches, sleep disturbances, depression, anxiety, memory loss, and difficulty concentrating, all of which can often be attributed to other factors as well. You might consider lowering your levels of exposure by keeping these items out of the bedroom and by turning off your cellular phone and MP3 player and unplugging electronic devices when not in use. Err on the side of caution: Charge your phone in the living room as opposed to the bedroom.

Chemical fire retardants known as polybrominated diphenyl ethers (PBDEs) are used in electronic consumer products and can also be toxic. PBDEs are also found in kitchen appliances, fans, hair dryers, and water heaters. To reduce exposure, use these machines in well-ventilated areas.

Last, check your home for mold. Cognitive symptoms associated with mold exposure include difficulty concentrating, irritability, brain fog, and memory changes. These symptoms have been correlated with one strain known as *Stachybotrys,* which is a green-black mold that grows on materials that contain cellulose, such as wood, paper, or drywall. Other molds that grow on tiles or cement can cause allergic reactions that can also affect your thinking.

Detox Your Home in Five Easy Steps

By following these suggestions, you'll reduce your sources of exposure and your body burden, and you may alleviate some of your symptoms.

1. Keep windows and doors open when cleaning so you don't trap air pollution inside.
2. Wear gloves for heavy-duty cleaning; cleansers, degreasers, and solvents can penetrate skin.
3. Check basements regularly for mold growth on walls, stored paper files, and books.
4. Remove dust by wiping floors and surfaces with a damp cloth instead of commercial dusting sprays.
5. A solution of one part vinegar to three parts water works just as well as potentially toxic commercial cleaners.

MEDICATIONS AND MEDICAL PROCEDURES CAN ADD TO YOUR BODY'S BURDEN

Recent advances allow for quick medical fixes, creating a culture where many people overtax their bodies and believe they can later reverse the damage through medications or surgery. At Canyon Ranch we believe it's always better to try to work on your lifestyle before you have to resort to medications or invasive procedures that can have detrimental side effects, especially in the brain, and that are often unnecessary.

The use of prescription medications is a good example. While they might relieve symptoms for one condition, they often have side effects that can cause a different problem, including changes in cognitive function. If you are taking medications and feel that your thinking is affected, speak with your doctor about possible side effects and other options that might be better for you. For instance, many people who take narcotics like codeine for pain find that their thinking seems sluggish. Antidepressants can improve mood, but can also cause suicidal thoughts. Each time you see your doctors, make sure they are aware of every medication you are taking, including over-the-counter remedies and herbal supplements; your doctors can help you avoid problems that can occur when medications are combined, or be able to sidestep unnecessary side effects entirely.

Some medications actually interfere with your innate ability to detoxify. Frequent use of acetaminophen, found in Tylenol, can deplete glutathione, a powerful antioxidant naturally produced in the body that is very important for detoxification. If you take acetaminophen daily, you may be depleting yourself of one of the most important substances your body needs to help you get rid of environmental toxins.

General anesthesia that accompanies a surgical procedure is considered to be safe; however, there have been reports showing that anesthesia may cause cognitive decline, especially in the elderly. Please keep this in mind if you are considering elective surgeries. This cognitive decline is called *postoperative cognitive dysfunction* (POCD), and it is still poorly understood. The risk of POCD increases with age and the condition occurs most frequently after cardiac surgeries, with a lower incidence after minor surgeries. Some researchers feel that it may be related to pre-operative stress, the administration of corticosteroids, or the mechanically induced circulation of blood. Patients with postoperative cognitive dysfunction report that they are more forgetful, have difficulty recalling words, and are often depressed. These changes are sometimes reversed, but often they are permanent. In one 2010 study, the progress of 270 patients over age sixty-five was followed after orthopedic surgery. After the first eight days, many patients showed early postoperative cognitive dysfunction in terms of their reaction time and ability to recognize three-dimensional objects. Thirteen months after surgery, many of the patients still had not recovered visuospatial functioning.

Toxic Foods

When guests come to Canyon Ranch, they frequently share with us how much they've learned about changing the way they eat. We feel that diet is one of the simplest yet most effective ways to make a significant change to your overall health, and particularly to your brain health. That's because the age-old saying "You are what you eat" is exactly true. Toxic foods are just as dangerous to your overall health, and particularly to your brain, as chemicals in the environment. Their affect is not sudden but cumulative.

You have to act as your own toxic-food detective and learn to recognize which foods are affecting your thinking. In chapter 6, we've outlined a four-week eating plan filled with nutritious foods that have additive value for your health. In this chapter, let's first focus on the toxic foods you need to avoid.

- *Commercially prepared meals and snacks:* Most fast foods and supermarket items that come "ready to eat" are considered to be processed foods, and some are healthier options than others. As a rule, try to stay away from high-sugar/white-flour combinations, such as cookies, pastries, store-bought cakes and pies, and sugar-laden cereals. Another reason why packaged foods should be avoided whenever possible is that many scientists consider the preservative monosodium glutamate (MSG) and the artificial sweetener aspartame (found in Equal, NutraSweet, and Canderel) to be within a class of chemicals known as *excitotoxins,* which are thought to exacerbate a host of neurological diseases, including Alzheimer's, dementia, and Parkinson's disease.

- *Foods that contain antibiotics and hormones:* Farm-raised animals have been treated with antibiotics and hormones to make them grow faster and larger. Unfortunately, these medications end up on our plates when we consume conventionally produced milk and other dairy products, beef, pork, lamb, veal, chicken, and eggs. They are thought to interfere with your health by possibly affecting your hormone balance, much like other endocrine disrupters. Look for the "rBGH free" designation on meat and dairy products; this term guarantees that there was no hormone administration.

Antibiotics can affect our intestinal microflora, diminishing the beneficial bacteria and creating additional opportunity for yeast overgrowth. This in turn can affect the immune system as well as the brain, because excessive yeast can cause brain fog and fatigue. And because of the transgenerational effect, the consumption of conventionally produced dairy and meat should be avoided particularly by women intending to become pregnant, as it might have a negative impact on the baby.

CANYON RANCH STRATEGIES
FOR DETOXIFICATION

A good detox is like a minivacation—a break in your usual routine during which you take care of your toxic load. We help our guests with detoxification using a general strategy that you can follow at home.

These suggestions not only help naturally lower your body burden, they are basic lifestyle changes that you should continue with for the long run. Within thirty days, you might be able to see changes in how you feel and how you think, including diminished fatigue, muscle aches, digestive problems, and brain fog.

The following techniques are directly related to all three of the major avenues of detoxification: digestion/elimination, breathing, and sweat. Overall, the most important detoxification goal is to have regular bowel movements once or twice a day, because that is the most efficient way for toxins to leave the body.

Exercise Regularly

Exercise improves detoxification in several ways. First, it helps you keep an optimal weight so that you will have less fat to store toxins. Exercise also helps to increase the production of the various liver enzymes involved in detoxification, making them more efficient. Last, you'll be sweating out more toxins with a vigorous exercise program. You'll find more information about exercise and its benefits in chapter 7.

Hydration

We sometimes joke that our motto at Canyon Ranch should be "The best solution to pollution is dilution." Your body is approximately 60 percent water. Because water is continuously used in nearly every life process, it's crucial to keep replenishing the supply. You need to drink six to eight 8-ounce glasses of clean water every day to increase the elimination of toxins through urination and sweat. Good hydration is also important for energy, for hunger management, and to prevent constipation: when you are well hydrated, you will be able to have more frequent bowel movements, making detoxification through digestion even more efficient. The most important indicator of your hydration status is the concentration of your urine. If it is clear or light yellow, you're probably well hydrated.

But not just any water will do. Make sure to drink filtered water whenever possible and use filtered water to wash fruits and vegetables and to make ice. Glass or stainless steel receptacles are the best choices for carrying drinking water outside your home. Hot or cold coffee and tea can be considered in your total consumption of water, and vegetables and fruit also contribute to your daily intake. Last, consult your physician regarding the optimal amount of water to consume if you have kidney problems or congestive heart failure.

Choose Foods That Benefit Detoxification

Approximately 20 percent of our water intake comes from foods, so choosing foods with high water content will naturally aid in the detoxification process. According to the American Dietetic Association, apples, carrots, grapefruit, watermelon, and lettuces are all excellent choices for this reason.

Foods high in fiber are equally important because fiber helps you have regular bowel movements. High-fiber foods also help regulate blood sugar and lower cholesterol—all important factors for brain health. If you believe you are affected by toxins, you need to make fiber the main staple of your diet, at least until your symptoms begin to resolve. Your consumption goal should be between twenty-five and thirty-five grams of fiber per day, which equals about twenty grams of fiber for every thousand calories you eat. But be warned, it's not easy to reach this goal: you'll need to choose foods high in fiber for breakfast, lunch, dinner, and every snack. High-fiber foods include nuts, seeds (such as flaxseeds), whole grains, oatmeal, green leafy vegetables, legumes, beans (such as lentils), and berries.

Cruciferous vegetables are another category of excellent detoxifiers. These include broccoli, cauliflower, Brussels sprouts, cabbage, and rutabaga, and can be eaten either cooked or raw to attain their positive effects. Leeks, onions, and garlic help detoxification by providing sulfur. And don't forget the antioxidants you'll need to bind those free radicals and lower oxidative stress. Choosing colorful fruits and vegetables and drinking plenty of green tea are two of the easiest ways to increase your intake of antioxidants. For detoxification, you'll need to eat six to eight servings of fruits and vegetables a day. Remember that a typical serving size is not one for one—for example, a large apple may actually count as two servings; a big bowl of salad may be three servings. The Massachusetts Institute of Technology quantifies a serving of fruit as the size of a small baseball and a serving of vegetables as the glass part of a typical lightbulb.

Supplements

Eating foods high in fiber and antioxidants is the best way to achieve detoxification, because you are also getting other nutrients in the process. However, most authorities believe that many of us are deficient in important vitamins due to our less-than-perfect eating habits. If you know that you are deficient, it may be a good idea to speak with a nutritionist who can suggest which supplements you may need to achieve the higher antioxidant levels required to lower oxidative stress.

If you don't get enough fiber from foods, consider using a fiber supplement as well. Many companies make different fiber products that you can take either in pill form or as a powder to add to water, fruit juices, shakes, or smoothies. Choose the one that you will be most comfortable using and that you find most enjoyable. Most important, speak with your doctor before you begin any type of supplement program.

Sauna

Spending time in a sauna will cause you to sweat out toxins through the skin. Consider using a sauna for twenty to fifty minutes once or twice a week. We do not recommend more than an hour at a time. Each time, follow these simple precautions:

- Avoid alcohol and medications that may impair sweating and produce overheating before and after a sauna.
- Avoid heavy meals two hours before a sauna.
- Cool down gradually afterward instead of entering a cold plunge pool.

- Don't take a sauna when you are ill, and if you feel unwell during your sauna, leave the room.
- Drink two to four glasses of cool water after each use of the sauna.

Lymphatic Massage

Lymph nodes are present throughout the body as a whole separate system that flows alongside major arteries and veins. This type of massage is very gentle. It stimulates the flow of lymph and helps remove toxins that are stagnating in different body tissues because of poor flow. Jumping on a trampoline is another effective way to increase lymphatic flow.

TRY AN ELIMINATION DIET

Many people have food sensitivities that are affecting their thinking. Food sensitivities are different from food allergies because they are not life threatening, but they are still very important to uncover. Oftentimes, people who have food sensitivities find that they are constantly fatigued and experience attention deficit, hyperactivity, brain fog, or difficulty focusing. They may also have gastrointestinal problems that affect their ability to detoxify.

One way to determine if you have food sensitivity is to follow an elimination diet. Elimination diets aren't easy, but they are effective. You'll be able to see a correlation between the foods you eat and the symptoms they produce. In general, we recommend speaking with a nutritionist before starting an elimination diet. Under the nutritionist's guidance, it is likely that, for four to six weeks, you will be avoiding the most common foods that cause sensitivities. These include dairy, gluten, eggs, sugar, and nightshade vegetables.

Afterward, add only one category of food back into your diet for a few days. For example, the first week following an elimination diet, you should reintroduce only dairy products. During that week, see if your symptoms return. If they do, then you'll know that you have a sensitivity to dairy and that you should avoid it going forward. If not, then you can continue to eat dairy, and add back gluten and watch for symptoms again. Continue until you've added back all the foods you initially eliminated and determined what was causing your problems.

FOODS TO CHOOSE, FOODS TO AVOID

Food Type	Choose	Avoid

PRODUCE	• Fresh and frozen, preferably organic vegetables and fruits
	• PLU codes that begin with a 9 indicate organic produce
	• Less-contaminated produce:
	    Onions
	    Corn
	    Pineapple
	    Avocado
	    Asparagus
	    Sweet peas
	    Mangoes
	    Eggplant
	    Cantaloupe
	    Kiwi
	    Cabbage
	    Watermelon
		• Fresh fruits and vegetables with PLU stickers that begin with an 8: these indicate genetic modification
		• The following "Dirty Dozen" are produce items that may be contaminated with toxins:
		    Apples
		    Celery
		    Strawberries
		    Peaches
		    Spinach
		    Nectarines
		    Grapes
		    Sweet bell peppers
		    Potatoes
		    Blueberries
		    Lettuce
		    Kale/collard greens

GRAINS Grains are less likely to be contaminated with pesticides, etc., than other foods. Therefore, it is not crucial to purchase organic grains, with the exception of canola and corn.	• Look for the word *whole* in front of any grain—e.g., whole wheat, whole rye, whole durum semolina flour. The exception is oats: rolled oats are whole oats. • Organic or nongenetically modified corn foods	• Refined flour and refined grains • Enriched white flour, wheat, unbleached flour, or any other grain or flour that does not specify *whole*.

Food Type	Choose	Avoid
DAIRY AND DAIRY ALTERNATIVES	• Nonfat/low fat organic milk, yogurt, cheese, and dairy alternatives • Organic is especially important for high-fat dairy products.	• Dairy products from cows treated with hormones (such as recombinant bovine growth hormone, or rBGH) or antibiotics.

PROTEINS	• Lean proteins:
	  Wild fish
	  Shellfish
	  Canned light tuna or salmon
	  Beef and lamb
	  Pork
	  Chicken
	  Eggs
	• Meat:
	  Choose grass-fed over grain-fed
	  Choose organic over conventionally raised
		• Meat with additives/preservatives (e.g., cold cuts preserved with nitrates)
		• Meat from animals treated with antibiotics or hormones
		• Large fatty fish like tuna and swordfish

Wash Produce Properly

Produce may contain pesticide/herbicide residues, bacteria, and other microbes that need to be washed off. Use one teaspoon of mild soap in one gallon of water or purchase a prepared vegetable wash solution such as Environné (800-282-WASH, www.vegiwash.com) or Fit Fruit & Vegetable Wash (800-FIT-WASH, www.tryfit.com) to wash produce. Use a vegetable brush on hard produce whose skin you plan to eat. Peel wax-coated nonorganic produce. Always clean produce before cutting. Discard the outer leaves of cabbage and head lettuce.

WHAT EFFECT DOES FOOD HAVE?

The following components required for detoxification are present in these food choices:

Beneficial Food Component	Food Sources
B vitamins	Beans, whole grains, dark green leafy vegetables, orange juice
Thiols (sulfur)	Onions, garlic, crucifers, avocado, mushrooms
Glutathione	Cysteine: red peppers, garlic, onions, broccoli, Brussels sprouts, oats, and wheat germ, with sulfur- and B-vitamin-containing foods
Flavonoids	Red/purple/black fruits, tomatoes, green and black teas, red wine, garlic, onions
Copper, manganese, selenium, zinc	Nuts, whole grains, low-fat dairy, green leafy vegetables
Sulforaphane and indole-3-carbinol (I3C)	Cruciferous vegetables
Carotenoids	Orange and yellow vegetables and fruits, dark green vegetables
Vitamin C	Citrus fruits, tomatoes, potatoes, bell peppers
Vitamin E	Almonds, wheat germ, cold-pressed extra virgin olive oil, avocado, nuts, soybean/tofu, sunflower seeds, olives
Coenzyme Q10	Fish, peanuts, soybeans, organ meats
Bioflavonoids	Citrus fruits
Polyphenols	Green tea, berries
Isoflavones	Soy foods
Curcumin	Turmeric
Catechins	Green tea
Ellagic acid	Red grapes
Probiotics	Yogurt containing live active cultures, kefir
Soluble fiber	Oatmeal, legumes, apples, pears, bran
Insoluble fiber	Berries, potato with skin, bran, whole grains, vegetables

For More information . . .

A great resource for more information on how toxins affect our lives is the Environmental Working Group. Its team of scientists, engineers, policy experts, and others research government data, legal documents, scientific studies, and their own laboratory tests to expose threats to public health and the environment, and to find solutions. The group's website, www.ewg.org, contains a wide range of information, from the latest research studies to the best practices on organic farming to removing toxins from your home/office to identifying the healthiest cosmetics and housewares.

MINIMIZING STRESS AIDS DETOXIFICATION

High levels of stress worsen the effect of toxins. Certain chemicals require the enzyme catechol-O-methyltransferase (COMT) for detoxification. This enzyme is also used to neutralize molecules of stress hormones known as catecholamines. If you are very stressed, the enzyme may be "too busy" with stress-induced catecholamines, and then may not have enough capacity to also process other compounds out of the body as efficiently.

Stress can also negatively affect your digestive tract, increasing your body burden by inducing leaky gut syndrome. In this disorder, the integrity of the intestinal lining is compromised, and bacterial toxins and food antigens, as well as other toxins, can more easily penetrate the intestinal lining and get into our system.

Most of all, realize that detoxification takes time. You will not notice a change to your thinking overnight. However, if you can stick with a sensible detoxification program, especially if you have tested positive for any of the toxins listed in this chapter, you'll slowly see lasting improvement. In the next chapter we'll explore the power that a good night's sleep has on the brain. When you can combine a clean, detoxified body with a well-rested mind, you can exponentially increase the possibilities of improving your cognition.

Chapter 5

SLEEP PROVIDES BRAINPOWER

We instinctively know that it's important to get a good night's sleep. But for most of us, this goal is elusive. In our fast-paced world, where we're constantly trying to cram in as much as we can every single day, sleep can feel like a waste of time—a guilty pleasure. And when we do have the opportunity to sleep, we don't want to sacrifice the end of the day when we can finally make time for ourselves. This trade-off of sleep for productivity is nothing new: it has affected our culture beginning with the invention of the lightbulb. As long as we've had the ability to extend the day, we've lost part of our night, and we have been sleeping an average of an hour and a half less than our great-grandparents.

Worse, even when we do make time for sleep, many of us have trouble. A whopping 64 percent of all Americans report that they don't get enough sleep. Half of us have difficulties sleeping at least a couple of times a week, and a third of us have problems every single night.

While scientists and researchers are uncovering the mysteries of the brain, they are also unraveling the importance of sleep. We now know that without the proper amount of sleep, your brain—and your body—may age prematurely. As the Harvard professor J. Allan Hobson so eloquently put it, "Sleep is of the brain, by the brain, and for the brain."

> ### The Brain Grows During Sleep
>
> During sleep the body releases hormones that are essential for healing and rejuvenating cells, including new brain cells created through neurogenesis. One of these is growth hormone, which is released by the pituitary gland, located just below the brain; greater quantities are released in men than in women. The brain chemical GABA both promotes sleep and helps to release growth hormone, so it is critical that the brain continues to produce enough of this powerful neurotransmitter.

LET ME SLEEP ON IT

When we don't get enough sleep, we typically feel more irritable, have a harder time focusing, and are not as productive. But until recently we didn't know why. Previously, we believed that the brain remains only somewhat busy during sleep, and we pointed to the dreams we remember, or the worrying that keeps us up, as signs of this activity. The latest imaging studies have found that major cross sections of the brain are very active during sleep. It is now thought that during sleep, the brain is busy creating more neuronal connections and increasing neuroplasticity. Studies suggest that sleep is critical for allowing the brain to synthesize information, including making connections between ideas, which also increases cognitive capacities. In short, when we sleep well the brain can decipher new memories effortlessly. When we don't have enough sleep, this process is disrupted and, consequently, so is our thinking.

When it comes to the brain, the request "Let me sleep on it" proves to be surprisingly accurate. Imagine that your memories are like a deck of playing cards. Every day, you have millions of sensory experiences that involve touch, taste, sight, smell, and sound. Each one of these experiences is broken down to its simplest form and is imprinted on a separate playing card as a short-term memory. For example, when you talk to a friend on the phone, you are creating a number of new short-term memory cards: a visual of what your friend looked like the last time you saw her (card 1), what the conversation was about this time (card 2), and your experience of holding the phone to your ear (card 3). Then during sleep, the brain shuffles through all the short-term memory cards made over the course of the day and consolidates them into experiences that become filed as long-term memories. The brain creates a *declarative memory*, which contains the consciously recalled facts and knowledge based on this experience. Studies show that newly learned memories—the cards you created that day—are reactivated during sleep, and further connections are made between them and your older memories. In this example, during sleep your brain would review the new phone experience and potentially connect it to all other experiences you've had with this friend, as well as all the other experiences you've had talking to people on the phone.

This constant creation of neuronal connections is one of the many ways we improve our cognitive and even physical abilities—for example, athletes who get good sleep perform better than those who do not. Test scores, behavior, and the ability to pay attention all increase with more hours of good sleep. So whether you are trying to understand complex math equations, improve fine motor skills, or develop a good jump shot, your brain needs sleep.

The Consequences of Sleep Debt

According to *Scientific American*, sleep debt is the difference between the amount of sleep you should be getting and the amount you actually get. Not only the hours but even the minutes lost every night increase this deficit. Studies show that lack of sleep raises cortisol levels, which contribute to increased stress. Even short-term sleep debt leads to a decline in brain health, including brain fog, impaired vision, and trouble remembering. In one 2008 study from the University of California, Berkeley, researchers found that sleep deprivation affected the retention of positive memories more than neutral or negative memories. Researchers think this is one reason why poor sleep can lead to mood disorders and depression: if you are having a hard time remembering the good parts of your life, it's easy to view your life as less meaningful.

When researchers look at performance tests given after just one night of sleep deprivation, the results clearly show impairment in terms of reaction time and memory recall. And with each additional sleepless night, these functions keep decreasing. Even though the results are clear, you still might perceive that you're doing just fine—but the detrimental impact happens early and persists, despite our perception.

The founder of the world's first sleep disorders clinic, Stanford University professor Dr. William Dement, created an experiment in the desert where people had to drive a car through a specific course. The drivers had to stay on the track and avoid obstacles that popped up in front of them, such as a picture of a child chasing a ball. One group of participants drank beer until they were tested as being legally drunk. The second group was kept awake for thirty-six hours. During the experiment, the people who were sleep deprived were just as impaired behind the wheel as the people who were drunk. What this means is that whatever little amount of sleep you think you've been getting away with, it's likely that you need more.

How Much Sleep Do We Need?

The recommended prescription for an adult is seven to nine hours of good sleep in one consolidated batch. The number of hours you require will fall within this normal part of the bell curve. Yet some healthy people need only six hours, while another small subset might require as much as ten. The bottom line is not actually the number. You want to achieve the sufficient quantity of sleep you need as well as improve the quality of sleep. If you get up at the same time every morning without setting an alarm, if you feel rested and refreshed, if your energy is pretty decent most of the day, and if it takes you more than ten minutes to fall asleep when you get into bed, you're probably meeting your sleep needs. But if you have to hit the snooze button a few times every morning before you stagger out of bed, and at the end of the day you fall asleep in front of the TV, you are not getting enough sleep.

And while our sleep needs change from infancy through young adulthood, once we hit our twenties they remain stable for the rest of our lives. Unfortunately, it's our sleeping skills that generally decline. With age we awaken more easily in the middle of the night. We also learn to tolerate sleepiness and cope with poor sleep by making behavioral changes like drinking coffee or loading up on simple carbs to keep us energized throughout the day.

The food choices you make are possibly linked to the sleep you had the night before. Just two nights of sleep deprivation can change hormone levels, including the levels of hormones that regulate eating patterns. With poor sleep, the levels of the hormone cortisol increase (signaling the body to eat) while another hormone, leptin, which tells us when we are full, decreases. When these triggers are upset, we may be more likely to look for foods that provide energy. Yet these compensation strategies can never fully erase a sleep debt: you're better off relearning how to get more, better sleep than subsisting on doughnuts, energy drinks, and coffee.

> **Start Wishing You Were a Teenager**
>
> The old saying "sleeping like a baby" is not the goal. Instead, let's try to sleep like teenagers, because they are the best sleepers. They fall asleep easily, they stay asleep, they're hard to arouse, and they actually get more sleep overall than both babies and adults. Teens really need nine or more hours of sleep every night, but because they look and sometimes act like grownups, we often don't allow them the sleep they need.

WHAT'S HAPPENING WHILE YOU SLEEP

Every night we experience three stages of quiet sleep: N1 (drowsiness), N2 (light sleep), and N3 (deep sleep). Unless something disturbs the process, you will proceed smoothly through the quiet sleep cycle. In making the transition from wakefulness into light sleep, you spend only a few minutes in stage N1 sleep, but your body and brain change rapidly. An electroencephalogram (EEG)—a noninvasive brain-wave test just like an electrocardiogram for the heart—will show that the predominant brain waves slow to four to seven cycles per second, a pattern called theta waves. Body temperature begins to drop, muscles relax, and eyes often move slowly from side to side. During stage N1 sleep you begin to lose awareness of your surroundings, but can be easily jarred awake.

The N2, or *light sleep,* stage is really the first phase of true sleep. During this stage, your eyes are still and your heart rate and breathing slow down. Meanwhile, brief bursts of brain activity called *sleep spindles* occur, as brain waves speed up for roughly half a second or longer. Some researchers believe that sleep spindles play a role in consolidating declarative memories. EEG tracings also show a brain wave pattern called a *K-complex,* which represents an internal vigilance system that allows you to awaken if necessary.

Stage N3, or *deep sleep,* occurs as the brain becomes less responsive to external stimuli, making it difficult to awake. During this stage, large, slow delta waves are evident on an EEG. Breathing becomes more regular. Blood pressure falls, and pulse rate slows to about 20 to 30 percent below the waking rate. Blood flow is directed less toward your brain, which cools measurably. Right before this stage ends, the muscles that allow you to be upright against gravity become paralyzed, and this paralysis prevents you from acting out your dreams. However, there are some sleep disorders—like sleepwalking and sleep eating—in which this change doesn't occur. A loss of sleep during this stage may play a role in reducing daytime creativity, mood, and fine motor skills.

These three stages of quiet sleep alternate with periods of active sleep, which is referred to as REM, or *rapid eye movement.* During this time the body is still but the mind is racing. Your eyes dart back and forth behind closed lids. Your blood pressure increases, and your heart rate and breathing speed up to daytime levels. The sympathetic nervous system, which is responsible for monitoring the fight-or-flight response, may be more active during REM sleep as compared to when you're awake.

Dreaming also occurs during REM sleep. Many people don't

remember their dreams unless they wake up right after dreaming. Yet each of us has from three to five cycles of REM sleep per night, occurring every 90 to 120 minutes. The first such episode usually lasts only a few minutes, but REM time increases progressively over the course of the night. The final period of REM sleep may last a half hour. During this time the brain is focusing on learning and memory. Scientists believe that REM sleep restores the mind, perhaps by clearing out irrelevant information. Research has also focused on REM sleep and its critical role in the consolidation of *procedural memory*—the remembering of "how" to do something. One study from the Weizmann Institute of Science in Israel measured how well participants who had learned a new task improved their scores after a night's sleep. If they were prevented from having REM sleep, the improvements were lost. On the other hand, if they were awakened an equal number of times from quiet sleep, the improvements in scores were unaffected.

Each time you move from quiet sleep to REM sleep, you are completing a sleep cycle. For optimal brain health, you need a balance of the different types of sleep throughout the night. So if you are shorting yourself by ninety minutes or more of sleep, you are losing the equivalent of one entire sleep cycle, and one opportunity to improve memory and repair the brain. So in terms of overall brain health, the goal is to make the most of every cycle you have access to.

It's not unusual to be awake briefly at the end of one cycle before you drop into the next one, but most of the time even if you do wake up, you won't even realize it. However, part of the problem with insomnia is that you become aware of the fact you're awake, and you start worrying that you won't be able to fall back asleep. This is especially true when you first go to sleep. Each night, there is a four-hour critical window: you may notice that between the hours of 10:00 p.m. and 2:00 a.m. you get some of your best sleep. This is because these first few hours go toward paying back your sleep debt. Also, it may be harder to go back to sleep if you wake up after that four-hour period, because you no longer have the sleep debt that was making you tired in the first place.

UNDERSTANDING YOUR
CIRCADIAN RHYTHM

Another aspect of sleepiness is the *circadian rhythm,* our internal clock that controls the daily ups and downs of biological patterns, including body temperature, blood pressure, and the release of hormones. The brain's hypothalamus regulates the circadian rhythm in conjunction with the source of cellular energy, *adenosine triphosphate,* or ATP. When adenosine levels build to a critical amount, you're ready to go to sleep.

The word *circadian* means "about a day," and though the pattern is largely self-regulating, it responds to several external cues—including light—to keep it set at twenty-four hours. It regulates the times we remain awake, and balances them with the time we spend sleeping. Throughout the day, our energy ebbs and flows along with these opposing forces—however, we've learned to acclimate to factors that allow us to be daytime as opposed to nocturnal creatures, so we've suppressed the daytime sleep drive. There is growing information about persistent circadian rhythm mismatches being one culprit behind insomnia. Having a routine of when you are most likely to go to sleep and when you need to be up in the morning is the best way to reset your circadian rhythm.

The circadian rhythm makes your desire for sleep strongest between midnight and dawn, and to a lesser extent in midafternoon. In societies where taking a siesta is the norm, people are responding to this rhythm with a one- to two-hour afternoon nap during the workday and a correspondingly shorter sleep at night. Circadian rhythm may also shift as we get older. Young kids wake up at the crack of dawn and will crash early in the evening. But once they hit puberty, their internal clocks change, and they become night owls.

> **Sleep Cycles Versus Circadian Rhythms**
>
> Sleep cycles are different from circadian rhythms because they are within a sleep period, whereas the circadian rhythm takes place within a twenty-four-hour period.

> ### Don't Let a Good Nap Ruin Your Night
>
> Napping is great if it's restorative and doesn't interfere with your ability to fall asleep later at night. But if you find that it's throwing off your circadian rhythm, forgo it until your sleep is restored. If you have to nap, do a power nap: twenty to forty minutes at most.

WHY AREN'T YOU SLEEPING?

Now that you understand why you need to sleep, and what good sleep is, let's look at some of the biggest reasons why you may be having problems. Sometimes, simply reversing the following illnesses or conditions will help you achieve better sleep patterns and resolve your sleep debt. It's interesting to note that while these are all considered to be conditions of the body, it's clear that they are also directly affecting your brain health.

Obstructive Sleep Apnea

Obstructive sleep apnea (OSA) is one of the major causes of sleep deprivation. It occurs when you have a blockage or obstruction in the nasal cavities or throat or have a floppy tongue, which is obstructing your airways either partially or completely during the night. These issues can be caused by an anatomical obstruction or excessive weight gain. The obstructions deprive the brain and the body of oxygen and cause an automatic response that wakes you up just enough so that you breathe again, although you may not wake to the point of consciousness.

These upsets can occur all night long, yet people with sleep apnea very often have no clue. Instead, they'll wake up in the morning without feeling refreshed. Other subtle clues include waking up with a dry mouth or having to repeatedly go to the bathroom in the middle of the night. Many people with sleep apnea snore, but not all of them. And not all snoring is considered to be sleep apnea. Your partner might be a better detective than you in determining if you are suffering from sleep apnea: if you snore and are tired despite adequate sleep time, or if you have been told that you hold your breath during the night, you may be affected.

The proportion of people in the country who have sleep apnea is small—about 5 percent—but this number may be misleading. Typically, people tested for sleep apnea are those who are thought to be high risk. However, one group of researchers tested everyone who came to a small family practice clinic, regardless of health history or current symptoms. The study showed that 17 percent of the women and 33 percent of the men had some degree of sleep apnea. In fact, 54 percent of people with environmental allergies have enough upper airway resistance to interfere with their sleep.

You can have sleep apnea and not appear to be affected by it because we learn to make behavioral modifications during the day. Or your positive mood or levels of stress can keep you awake and energized. However, sleep apnea affects not only the quality and quantity of your sleep but also your brain. Cognitive problems, such as deficits in memory, attention, and visual abilities, frequently accompany OSA. A study from the Sungkyunkwan University School of Medicine in Seoul, Korea, showed that those suffering from OSA may have significantly reduced gray matter volume in the hippocampus, frontoparietal cortices, temporal lobe, anterior cingulate, and cerebellum. This may suggest neuronal cell loss as well as cognitive decline during wakefulness, including memory impairment.

Obstructive sleep apnea also affects your body's health. It is a major risk factor for heart disease and stroke, since as many as two-thirds of people with underlying sleep apnea have high blood pressure. In fact, people who've had a stroke and who suffer from untreated sleep apnea are 4.5 times more likely to have another stroke. If you are periodically depriving your blood of oxygen, the blood vessels will become more spastic as they try to keep blood flowing. Over time, the vessels may lose their elasticity, and inelasticity leads to hypertension.

Diabetes

More and more research suggests that sleep deprivation actually makes us hungrier, more stressed, and more resistant to insulin. All of these conditions can lead to type 2 diabetes. We also know that people with high blood sugar have sustained damage to their small blood vessels and nerves, which can cause pain during sleep, including neuropathy in the legs.

Sleep apnea also coexists with diabetes. As many as 55 to 85 percent of people with diabetes may also have sleep apnea. Data suggest that sleep apnea may actually precipitate the development of diabetes, because after as little as two weeks, short-term sleep deprivation can overstimulate your production of hormones, insulin, and glucose. Luckily, when people with diabetes get treated for sleep apnea, they may find that their weight, blood pressure, cholesterol levels, and sugars go down, because they are remedying the underlying problem.

Depression

There are classic sleep patterns that are part of the diagnostic criteria for depression. The most common is waking up in the early morning hours and being unable to go back to sleep. Another one is referred to as *hypersomnolence,* which means the desire or need to sleep all the time. Other components of depression include feeling helpless, hopeless, and sad.

It is unclear if sleeplessness causes depression, or if depression leads to a lack of sleep. Some researchers believe it is both. Multiple studies have shown that when people with no prior history of depression are subjected to sleep deprivation, it often can cause the development of depression, postpartum depression, and even suicidal thoughts.

Fibromyalgia

A high percentage of people with fibromyalgia have abnormal sleep patterns. Fibromyalgia is characterized by widespread pain areas, fatigue, sleep disturbance, and often problems with cognition, such as brain fog. Fibromyalgia is often diagnosed after blood tests have ruled out other possible diagnoses.

However, what do you think happens to healthy people when you shortchange their sleep for a week? By the end of the week, three-quarters of them can have developed some sort of achy pain syndrome, headaches, achy joints, or stiffness. You might find that you get relief from these symptoms if you can restore proper sleep patterns.

Attention Deficit Disorder

Not everyone with ADD has a sleep disorder; however, we do know that getting a good night's sleep can naturally help us stay alert and focused. We also know that someone with ADD will have more attention difficulties the day after a night of poor sleep.

Reflux

Reflux occurs when the acid in the stomach splashes back into the esophagus. Gravity can play a role, and many people find that they experience more reflux when they are lying down at night. Unfortunately, this can affect your sleep patterns: reflux can cause you to wake up in the middle of the night with a cough because the acid travels into the lungs. You can also wake up feeling hoarse.

Restless Legs

The phrase *restless legs* describes the irresistible urge to move when you are sitting quietly or lying down, most commonly at nighttime. Sometimes it can just be an abnormal sensation, or it can be accompanied by muscle twitching. For some people these urges to move can affect the entire body, causing thrashing, flailing, or constant movement. And because all this activity occurs at night, it can clearly affect your sleep. Interestingly, movement disorders like this don't begin in the arms or legs; they begin in the brain. They are related to a lack of production of the neurotransmitter dopamine, and they may be treated with the same medications used to treat Parkinson's disease. Movement disorders also may be related to a lack of iron in the diet—your brain needs iron to make dopamine.

Hormone Loss

Even if you're not having hot flashes, you may be experiencing hormonal decline. This is true for both men and women, because each of us produces all three sex hormones: estrogen, progesterone, and testosterone. Estrogen is necessary for maintaining sleep once you fall asleep, and progesterone makes you drowsy, so when these levels decline, your circadian rhythm may be disrupted. Progesterone is also a respiratory stimulant, and a loss seems to correlate with the onset of sleep apnea. This may be one reason why older adults suffer from sleep apnea, or why sleep becomes a problem as we get older. For example, pregnant women don't typically have more sleep apnea, even though they have gained weight, but their progesterone levels are through the roof—they breathe faster, and their higher progesterone levels may be creating the mechanism so they can sleep.

Doctors sometimes prescribe hormone replacement therapies to resolve sleep issues. Low-dose bioidentical hormones may actually help restore sleep and improve the symptoms related to menopause that are preventing sleep from occurring in the first place, including hot flashes and depression.

Medications

There are many different medications that interfere with sleep. Steroids, decongestants, ADD medications, and beta blockers are common culprits. Antidepressants—particularly SSRIs, including Prozac, Zoloft, and Lexapro—can disrupt sleep, especially when you first start them or change the dosage.

Adequate pain control is important for a good night's sleep, and vice versa. Chronically painful conditions can also interfere with your quality of sleep. If you hurt because you've got arthritis, and every time you roll over in bed, you ache and it wakes you up, you can be caught in a cycle of pain and sleep disruption.

The Truth About Insomnia

Primary insomnia is very rare. For most of us, poor sleep is a response to a trigger around which we developed a thought pattern. We wake in the middle of the night and start going through our list of worries. Then we start to worry and get anxious about losing sleep, and it develops into a different, more complicated pattern.

CANYON RANCH SLEEP STRATEGIES

Guests at Canyon Ranch often ask, "When I can't get to sleep, should I just lie there and close my eyes? Can I meditate? Or should I just get out of bed and do something else?" The truth is, there's no replacement for sleep.

At the ranch, we work with guests to figure out what's keeping them up at night, and then teach them how to reset their lifestyle so they can consistently achieve a better night's sleep. These suggestions are the first line of defense, and for the most part they are easy fixes you can make in your home and in your bed so you can get the rest your brain needs to function better tomorrow.

Try any and all of the following until you find something that's just right for you.

Get Out of Bed

If you wake up in the middle of the night and you can't go back to sleep, you need to break whatever cycle you've learned or adopted that keeps you up and worrying. Without turning on too much light, get out of bed and read a book. Or go into another room and do something calming until you're sleepy again and can come back to bed.

Sleep restriction is a specific technique that can address difficulty in getting to sleep once you are in bed. The goal is to promote sleep efficiency. The technique is based on the assumption that sleep deprivation will increase the drive to sleep and to remain asleep. It will also help reset your brain so that you will connect your bed with the idea of sleep. By limiting the amount of time in bed to approximately the amount of time spent sleeping, you make the bed a conditioned stimulus for sleep. Over several nights this technique can have a dramatic impact and often results in significant improvement in the quality and quantity of sleep.

For the week prior to starting the sleep restriction technique, record what time you attempted to go to sleep and how many hours you slept. Once you determine an average amount of total sleep, choose a time that you can commit to being awake each morning. Your waking time must be constant, so do not begin this program if you will be traveling, vacationing, or on a deadline for a project.

Once you are ready to begin, you will limit the amount of time in bed to close to the average number of hours usually slept. For example, if your sleep journal shows that you are sleeping only five hours a night, you will allow yourself only five hours into bed. Set your alarm clock for your waking time, and then work backward by adding five hours to determine what time you need to enter the bed.

It may be necessary to use light physical activity to stay up until the scheduled bedtime. You might want to avoid sitting in front of a TV if in the past you have had a tendency to fall asleep on the couch, only to find yourself lying awake after getting into bed. In the hour or so before bedtime, begin to wind down by engaging in relaxing activities such as listening to music or doing the relaxation techniques listed later in this chapter.

After a few nights, move your bedtime back by about thirty minutes a week until an optimal amount of sleep is reached. Once you find that your awakenings have been reduced and no further improvement is gained by going to bed earlier or sleeping later, an optimal bedtime and rise time will have been determined.

Adjust the Noise

We get used to the ambient noise that accompanies our lives. People who live in the city often have a hard time sleeping at Canyon Ranch because it's too quiet. And when people leave the ranch and return to their lives, they can have the opposite problem. White noise machines can be helpful when you are transitioning from one place to another, because they drown out the ambient noise of a new environment and provide a steady, consistent amount of noise, which you can become conditioned to and which will help you fall asleep.

Shut Off All Lights

The optic nerves are some of the most responsive and the quickest to cause arousal. This is one of the reasons why it's hard to sleep in the bright sun. Additionally, the pineal gland, which secretes the hormone melatonin that helps induce drowsiness, is also sensitive to light. You may need to invest in new window shades that keep your room dark, or cover your eyes with a sleep mask, because even the smallest amounts of light emitted from an alarm clock, the TV, a computer, or a smartphone can wreak havoc on sleep.

I once met a woman who was excited to tell me about her new bedroom clock. "It shines the time on the ceiling, so if I wake up, I don't have to roll over and look at my clock to know what time it is." My advice was to cover up the alarm clock at night and make sure her room was really dark. Then I explained that there is no real reason why she should need to know the time in the middle of the night. The truth is, you need to know what time it is only when it's time to get up, because in the middle of the night this knowledge automatically starts a thought process: "It's two a.m. Why am I awake?"

In fact, all these tiny blinking lights can add up to real annoyances at bedtime. One sleep researcher from the University of Chicago raised concerns about people using mobile phones, e-readers, and iPads as reading sources before going to bed. He made the obvious connection that the direct light they emit may interfere with your ability to fall asleep. What's more, they provide easy access to reviewing emails and text messages before bed, which in and of itself stimulates the brain. Instead, we suggest that you create a different, less electronically focused ritual that separates your sleep from the rest of the day.

Turn Down the Thermostat

The best environment for sleeping is a room with low humidity that's nice and cool. You might think you're treating yourself if you buy luxurious down comforters, but if you are too hot at night, you might not be able to sleep peacefully. Another way to cool down before bed is to take a warm, but not hot, shower. Your body is less rambunctious when it's cooler. Not only will the shower relax the body; it can help create a new sleep ritual, separating your daytime events from sleep.

Children, Pets, and Bed Partners

Young children love to crawl into their parents' bed, but letting your child sleep there through the night may cause difficulties for your sleep as well as the child's. First, remember that children's sleep cycles aren't the same as yours. Second, their breathing and restlessness can interfere with your comfort. The same is true if you have a cat nuzzled at your neck and the family dog sleeping on top of your feet.

The problem becomes exponentially more difficult if your spouse or partner is what's keeping you awake. If your partner snores or is restless—pulling the covers off and thrashing around in bed—or is on a different schedule, your sleep will suffer. As with all aspects of a good relationship, honesty is the best policy. Sit down and strategize how to make adjustments that work for both of you. Otherwise, you have to realize that your lack of sleep is making your relationship more difficult than it needs to be. When you're sleep deprived, you'll feel more anxious, more irritable, angrier, and more resentful.

If your partner snores, he or she needs a sleep study (which is described below). We find that time after time, when you treat one member of a couple, both benefit. You might also want to consider setting up a sleep schedule. One couple I know sleep together two nights a week, and then separately on other nights. Others manage using headphones or earplugs. The bottom line is that you shouldn't give up your sleep for your relationship, or the other way around.

Reduce Overstimulation and Stress

Stress and anxiety are often the reasons why it's hard to fall asleep in the first place, or why it's hard to get back to sleep when you wake up. The mind starts going and you can't shut it off. In fact, anxiety is often more prevalent at night because during the day you can block out your worries when you are busy with other things. At night, there are no more distractions, and your worries can come flooding in.

Behavioral therapists recommend setting a small part of the day aside as "worry time," when you can run through the things that are bothering you. Others find that keeping an evening journal is a good strategy for addressing stressors. Either technique allows you to deal with your problems instead of ignoring them. You're also giving yourself an outlet, and you're paying attention to your problems, so hopefully you can use this space to resolve these issues. Once they are compartmentalized, you can put them aside so that they are not in the forefront of your thoughts as you're trying to sleep.

In my home, I have a notepad on my nightstand. If I wake up in the middle of the night and I'm plagued by a worry, I don't turn on the light. Instead, I'll reach for my notepad and just jot something down. Then I can get back to these thoughts in the morning and address whatever was threatening to keep my brain busy.

Last Call for Caffeine and Skip the Nightcap

If you have to get up multiple times in the middle of the night to empty your bladder, you will disrupt your sleep cycle. We recommend that you stop drinking beverages of all types about two hours prior to your bedtime.

If you're having a tough time falling asleep at ten o'clock at night, think back to when you had your last cup of coffee. The half-life of caffeine can be as long as seven to eight hours, which means that for some people, the 8:00 a.m. cup of coffee is still affecting their system at 10:00 p.m., even though only a quarter of a cup is left in their system.

Some people can tolerate a quarter of a cup, but for others, even that minute amount will affect their sleeping.

You may have a pretty good sense of where you are in that spectrum. Some people can have an espresso and go right to bed. Others will drink a cup of coffee, feel wired and anxious, and be unable to sit still the rest of the day. That latter type probably metabolizes foods more slowly.

Last, think about your patterns with alcohol. Many people find as they get older that after they have a couple of drinks, they fall right asleep, only to find themselves wide awake a few hours later. This is a very typical pattern because it takes a couple of hours for you to process the sugars found in alcohol, and once they clear your system, you wake up. For every drink you have, you get one hour of sedation followed by one hour of arousal. So if you have a nightcap, it might put you to bed at first, but then it may disrupt your sleep afterward.

Alcohol also relaxes the tissues that hold your airway open, making you more prone to sleep apnea. Keep in mind that both alcohol and coffee are notorious hot-flash triggers and bladder irritants. You may actually be giving yourself a triple whammy with regard to your sleep quality if you're a perimenopausal woman who consumes caffeine and alcohol late in the daytime and into the evening.

You might want to stay clear of both caffeine and alcohol until your sleep patterns have normalized. Then you can reintroduce one at a time and notice how they affect your sleep and your thinking. You may realize you can tolerate one cup of coffee as long as it's before 10:00 a.m., but if you have a second cup in the afternoon, it will keep you awake. In short order you'll be able to find what works for you and what doesn't.

Make Better Food Choices Before Bedtime

Your digestive tract is not supposed to be working hard at night. It's supposed to be resting, so you don't want to have a big meal before you go to bed. While a full stomach can make you tired, it can also cause heartburn, which can make your sleep uncomfortable and trigger arousal during the night. In general, finish eating a large meal least two or three hours before bedtime.

The flip side of this is that a light, complex-carbohydrate-rich meal may actually boost production of the brain chemicals serotonin and melatonin, both of which relax the brain and help you sleep. A glass of milk is a good source of tryptophan, which is one of the building blocks of protein that is known to make you feel sleepy. This is why some people find that a light snack of complex carbohydrates—such as a small bowl of cereal—at bedtime may actually help them fall asleep. Check serving sizes to make sure you are not eating too much before bedtime, and remember to brush your teeth afterward; milk has lots of natural sugars that can cause cavities if they are left sitting in your mouth overnight.

Keep in mind that an overtired brain is a hungrier brain. If you are constantly fatigued, you're more likely to overeat the next day and to make poor food choices at night.

Invest in a Comfortable Mattress

If you've been sleeping on the same mattress for more than ten years, it's time to buy a new one. Shop around to find one that is comfortable for you and your partner. It doesn't matter if it is firm or soft as long as you feel supported. And don't buy into the latest fads: go for comfort. Those memory foam beds sound really nice but are known to pack in body heat and may not be the best choice for premenopausal or menopausal women.

Then choose bedding that breathes. Pillow density is a personal preference, but cotton sheets, blankets, and comforters will let air circulate over you, keeping you cooler at night. Choose colors that don't overstimulate your senses; muted colors and sheets that are soft to the touch are the best options.

Change Your Sleep Position

Sometimes, shifting off your back may be all you need to ensure a better night's sleep. Sleeping on your back may exacerbate sleep apnea because your tongue falls back and blocks your airway. Side sleepers may snore less, with the result that not only will you sleep better, so will your partner.

Exercise During the Day, Meditate at Night

The areas of the brain that sleep the best are those that are the most active during the day. Many people notice that when they come to Canyon Ranch they sleep better because they are so physically active during the day. The timing of exercise is also important: you may find that if you engage in aerobic activity too close to bedtime, you feel so energized that you can't go to sleep.

Instead, develop a relaxation practice that can include meditation, light stretching, or even some yoga postures to help you fall asleep. Simply slowing down your breathing can harness a relaxation response. You'll learn more about breathing techniques and meditation in chapter 8.

TREATING CHRONIC SLEEP PROBLEMS

If the suggestions above are not enough to make a significant difference in your sleep, the following are the next steps in good care. These suggestions require that you visit at least your own doctor, if not a specialist.

Investigate with a Sleep Study

If you are giving yourself the opportunity for sleep yet constantly feel fatigued or have any of the physical conditions described earlier in the chapter, regardless of whether you have been told that you snore, you probably ought to participate in a sleep study. This test is typically given by a sleep specialist or an ENT (ear, nose, and throat doctor).

During a sleep study you are asked to spend the night in a special room, which may be at an outpatient sleep center or in a medical center or hospital. You sleep in your own clothing, and the administrator applies monitors to the head, chest, abdomen, arms, and legs. A sleep specialist may also consider a portable study that can be completed in your home. With either type of test, you are able to get your results quickly, often the next day. Sleep studies are accurate for the night they are performed—they cannot predict what happens every night—but if you replicate a typical night's sleep during the study, it will be the most effective.

A sleep study tests your brain waves, eye movements, heart rate, obstructions to breathing patterns, and overall body movement. The brain waves and eye movements will show which stage of sleep you are having difficulty with. It will also definitively show you on video if you are actually sleeping through the night or if you are suffering from nighttime seizures or something as simple as lying in an uncomfortable sleep position. An oxygen meter provides basic information as to your breathing and how well you are moving air in terms of the mouth, nose, and chest.

Treating Sleep Apnea

The standard treatment for sleep apnea uses a device referred to as *continuous positive airway pressure* (CPAP), a mask you wear over your nose and mouth that is hooked up to a machine to make sure you have a constant supply of air during the night. CPAP provides a column of air to prevent the airway from collapsing or creating an obstruction. An added benefit of the CPAP machine was highlighted in a 2011 study published in the *Journal of the American Medical Association*, which showed that those who use it who suffer from both sleep apnea and mild cognitive impairment can improve their memory and reduce attention loss. It may also help lower the risk of developing dementia by improving oxygen flow.

Many people are initially scared of wearing the mask, especially if they are claustrophobic. However, the mask is so effective that once you get used to wearing one, you may not be able to sleep without it. What's more, sleep specialists can make small adjustments to the masks to make them more comfortable to wear; such adjustments help most people consistently use their CPAP if they are motivated to do so.

Behavioral Therapy

For some people, getting into the pattern of having a good night's sleep is really a matter of addressing thought patterns we've developed about what it means to be in bed and getting to sleep. There are many possible goals of behavioral therapy—among the most common is to shift the anxiety about being in bed and not being able to fall asleep into something more productive. Cognitive behavioral therapy (CBT) can address these and other issues in as little as one or two sessions. It can also take as long as several months. However, research has noted the clear benefits of this work toward improving insomnia and promoting a better night's rest.

CBT allows you to analyze the problems that are making it hard for you to sleep and change your behaviors to deal with these problems. The process typically involves a therapist who will employ any of the following techniques:

- Good sleep hygiene: using good sleep habits, such as staying on a sleep schedule
- Psychotherapy: helping you to remove the thoughts that are keeping you awake
- Relaxation techniques
- Sleep diaries
- Stimulus control therapy: removing the factors that are causing your mind to resist going to sleep

Other behavioral techniques include sleep restriction, which we discussed earlier, as well as relaxation techniques such as those found in chapter 8. One Canadian study reported in the *Journal of the American Medical Association* tested people with insomnia using sleeping pills, cognitive behavioral therapy, or a combination. The group that did the best was actually the cognitive behavioral therapy group. Behavioral treatment, singly or combined, was rated by subjects, significant others, and clinicians as more effective than drug therapy alone. Subjects were also more satisfied with the behavioral approach.

Medications

Sleep aids are meant to help the mind and body relax so you can fall asleep and stay asleep. They are not a cure for insomnia. They are, however, enormously popular, especially because the United States allows pharmaceutical companies to advertise directly to the public.

At Canyon Ranch, we do not promote prescription sleep medications as the first line of defense against sleep disorders. However, we recognize that for some people they do offer relief. Sometimes people use them when they're traveling to a new time zone—they'll take an Ambien to get to sleep at the desired time. Sleep medications have also been proven to be beneficial for people newly diagnosed with sleep apnea.

These medications provide short-term relief, working as part of a behavioral modification program. In fact, most studies showing their efficacy were conducted over periods ranging from only six to eight weeks. However, many people start taking sleeping pills and stay on them for years. Unfortunately, there aren't many long-term studies that follow this type of usage. And while sleep medications supposedly do not cause physical addiction, in our experience at Canyon Ranch, we see many guests who have developed a psychological addiction to them: they become convinced they cannot sleep without them. Worse, some of these medications can lead to amnesia. There have been reports of people eating, driving, or cooking food in their sleep and having no recollection the next day.

Sleep medications are grouped by their scientific class, and some can be quite detrimental to the brain. The older medications include depressants, known as *barbiturates,* such as Amytal, Nembutal, and Seconal. These medications interfere with the sleep cycle, so when people take them, they fall asleep but do not achieve good-quality sleep. Antidepressants are also prescribed as a sleep aid, although these are thought to reduce REM sleep. *Benzodiazepines* are also commonly used medications in the treatment of insomnia. They are considered to be safer than some of the older barbiturate sleeping medications.

In recent years, a newer class of medications has been developed and is often referred to as *nonbenzodiazepine hypnotics*. These newer medications include Ambien, Sonata, and Lunesta and are used to reduce the time it takes to fall asleep. They appear to have better safety profiles and less adverse effects than earlier sleep medications. They are also associated with a lower risk of abuse and dependence. The most common side effects include daytime drowsiness, dry mouth, and dizziness.

Desyrel (trazodone) is most commonly used to treat depression, but it is the most prescribed off-label medication for sleep. There are very limited studies supporting its use and efficacy. Nevertheless, at Canyon Ranch we have seen some guests who have noted that it significantly reduced or eliminated their insomnia. Its main side effect is daytime sedation, along with the feeling of being hungover, constipation, dry mouth, grogginess, and urinary retention.

Don't Experiment with Sleep Meds

Never take someone else's medications, especially sleep meds. Even if these provide great relief for your best friend or your spouse, it's important to remember that we each have a distinct brain chemistry, and the particular sleep aid that was prescribed to someone else was meant to balance only that person's brain. What will work great for some might be a disaster for you. Instead, talk to your doctor to determine which medication best matches your health history and current health status.

The Most Commonly
Prescribed Sleep Aids

Trade Name	Generic Name	Common Side Effects
Ambien	Zolpidem	Dizziness, dry mouth
Ativan	Lorazepam	Hangover effect
Dalmane	Flurazepam	Hangover effect
Desyrel	Trazodone	Daytime sedation, urinary retention
Doral	Quazepam	Hangover effect
Halcion	Triazolam	Hangover effect
Klonopin	Clonazepam	Hangover effect
Lunesta	Eszopiclone or estorra	Dizziness, dry mouth
ProSom	Estazolam	Hangover effect
Restoril	Temazepam	Hangover effect
Sonata	Zaleplon	Dizziness, dry mouth
Xanax	Alprazolam	Hangover effect

Treating Pain So You Can Sleep

Pain and sleep have a particular chicken-and-egg relationship. Those in pain will have difficulty sleeping. And the person who doesn't sleep as much will be likely to hurt more. Unfortunately, many pain medications can harm the brain. Yet if you don't relieve your pain, you won't be able to sleep.

We've found that it's best to treat both pain and sleep together. The most common choices are low doses of *sedating antidepressants,* even for those with chronic pain who are not experiencing significant or clinical depression. The ones most commonly used include Desyrel (trazodone), Elavil (amitriptyline), and Sinequan (doxepin).

Over-the-Counter Sleep Aids and Herbal Supplements

Supplements and over-the-counter medications can be just as effective as prescription medications. They can also be just as dangerous. The fact that something's available without a prescription doesn't necessarily mean it's safe. Many of the following can interfere with your current health status, especially if you are already taking prescription medications. Discuss each of these options with your doctor before taking one of them.

Antihistamines: Allergy medications, such as Benadryl (diphenhydramine), cause many people to feel sleepy and are also very good at keeping you asleep. In fact, many over-the-counter sleep aids are simply the generic form of this medication. Look for the name diphenhydramine in the active ingredients list. Side effects can include constipation, impaired daytime functioning, urinary retention, and glaucoma risk (especially in the older adult).

Melatonin: This supplement is actually a hormone that can help you speed up the process of falling asleep. Melatonin is naturally produced in the brain. It circulates throughout the body in a daily cycle and is responsible for helping you maintain your circadian rhythm. It's often used by night-shift workers, and it is also good for travel, especially if you are changing time zones. When used correctly, melatonin is conducive to resetting the timing of your sleep cycle, thereby putting you to sleep, but it will not keep you asleep.

5-hydroxytryptophan (5-HTP): A chemical produced in the body from the nutrient tryptophan, which is found in foods including dairy products and turkey. When tryptophan is converted into 5-HTP, it is changed into the brain chemical serotonin, and then into melatonin. Supplements of 5-HTP therefore raise serotonin levels in the brain. This elevation can relax you, and is thought to have a positive effect on sleep, mood, anxiety, appetite, and pain sensation; however, people who are already taking anti-depressants or antianxiety medications that increase or reduce serotonin in the brain should avoid this option. In one study, people who took 5-HTP went to sleep more quickly and slept more deeply than those who took a placebo. However, it may take six to twelve weeks for the 5-HTP to be fully effective.

Magnesium: This essential mineral affects neuromuscular control. Certain medical conditions can upset the body's magnesium balance—for example, vomiting or diarrhea can cause temporary magnesium deficiencies. Too much coffee, soda, salt, or alcohol, as well as heavy menstrual periods, excessive sweating, and prolonged stress, can also lower magnesium levels. When you are deficient in magnesium, you may experience muscle spasms. Supplementing a deficiency may help relieve some of the discomfort associated with mild cases of restless leg syndrome. It can also help you wind down and fall asleep.

Hops: A plant that is most commonly used to improve the flavor of beer. Hops are also used as a treatment for anxiety, restlessness, and insomnia. Because they have a fragrant smell, they have been used as part of aromatherapy: a pillow filled with hops is a popular folk remedy for sleeplessness. Hops may be used alone, but more frequently they are combined with other herbs, such as valerian and lemon balm.

SUPPLEMENTS TO AVOID

Kava kava, also known simply as kava, is an herbal supplement thought to treat anxiety and relieve insomnia. However, numerous side effects are possible, and some are quite severe, including liver toxicity. For this reason, we agree with the National Institutes of Health and advise that you use kava only under the supervision of a health care practitioner.

St. John's wort is another herbal supplement thought to promote better sleep. However, it can limit the effectiveness of many prescribed medications such as blood thinners, birth control pills, and some anti-cancer medications.

For More Information . . .

One important aspect of the National Institutes of Health is the National Center for Complementary and Alternative Medicine. This organization is the federal government's lead agency for scientific research on these types of remedies. Its mission is "to define, through rigorous scientific investigation, the usefulness and safety of complementary and alternative medicine (CAM) interventions and their roles in improving health and health care." Its website, www.nccam.nih.gov, offers a wealth of research on the efficacy of different therapies. You can use this resource to begin having an educated conversation with your doctor to determine which supplements may be right for you.

• • •

Now that you understand some of the intricacies of the brain and how it can be affected by your current health and your environment, you can begin to explore easy and effective ways to reverse damage and increase cognitive function.

PART TWO

30 Days at the Ranch

Chapter 6

THE 30-DAY EATING PLAN—
MAXIMIZING BRAIN FUNCTION
THROUGH NUTRITION

When it comes to maintaining and even enhancing brain health, choosing the right foods is critically important. The latest studies have shown that the ability to retain healthy brain cells as well as increase the number of new cells and neuronal connections via neurogenesis is significantly influenced by the foods we eat every day. The quality of these brain cells is just as important as the quantity, and the choices we make at the table can either support brain function or work against it.

Caring for both body and mind through nutrition increases your potential for remaining intellectually engaged now and for years to come. What's more, an eating program filled with nutrient-rich, high-quality foods will increase your chances for avoiding some of the most common diseases that can affect brain health as well as your potential longevity: obesity, diabetes, and cardiovascular disease.

This chapter provides everything you need to know to make the best food choices that support brain health. This plan is not geared for weight loss, because building new brain cells requires eating plenty of the right foods. Consuming too few calories will actually starve the brain. When the brain starts to feel that it is getting low on fuel, it drives you to find a quick source in the form of carbohydrates; we experience this drive as food cravings. At the same time, the brain forces what we call a *starvation response,* which causes the immediate storage of food as body fat, so that it will be available to the brain at another time. This strategy works for the brain but not for the belly. However, you might find that by feeding your brain regularly and improving your food choices, you may also drop a few pounds.

You'll see that on this plan we're not going to ask you to make drastic changes to your diet: you won't have to go through the kitchen cabinets and throw everything out. Nor are we recommending a specific diet that everyone should follow—that simply isn't the Canyon Ranch way. We believe that every individual has specific needs based on genetics, medical history, health status, eating preferences, and lifestyle, and there is no such thing as a one-size-fits-all diet. What's more, we believe in making incremental modifications to the way you eat right now that will last a lifetime. Each week for the next four weeks, you'll learn how to make one simple change to your diet that can improve brain health.

The Last Word on Portion Control

The relationship between food quantity and overall aging is clear: less is better. When we overeat, we are actually causing injury at the cellular level, which hastens aging. In order to prevent that, you have to watch not only what you eat but how much you are eating.

Many Okinawans in Japan practice an ancient Confucian teaching called *Hara hachi bu,* which roughly translates as "Eat until you're 80 percent full." This guarantees that you won't overeat beyond what your body can safely process, digest, assimilate, and distribute, and you won't overwhelm the system. However, it's hard to quantify what 80 percent means, because that number is going to be different for each of us. What we can do is remain conscious of the fact that there always will be another meal coming down the pike. So if you finish 80 percent of whatever you are served, you can save the rest for a snack later in the day.

By the end of the month, you'll be able to pull these changes together, and your cumulative learning will be effortlessly incorporated into your daily dietary routine.

THE CANYON RANCH PHILOSOPHY OF HEALTHY EATING

Our philosophy is based on what we like to call *nutritional intelligence,* the integration of practical food and nutrition knowledge with an understanding of yourself. Developing your nutritional intelligence can lead to sustainable and effective eating strategies that meet your unique needs. Over the next thirty days, not only will you learn to eat to improve your brain health, you'll also learn how to identify when certain foods affect you mentally and physically, both positively and negatively.

The guiding principles of nutritional intelligence include:

Honor your individuality. Many factors influence your nutrient requirements—genetics, medical history, health status, eating preferences, lifestyle, and more. Acknowledge the various roles food and eating play in your life, and as you read through this chapter, determine if your existing relationship with food is healthy.

Practice engaged eating. Eating should be a joyful experience that engages your physical and emotional senses. Maximize your enjoyment of food by indulging your preferences for flavor and texture and by creating meaningful mealtime rituals. Eat slowly, chew thoroughly, and savor the sensual experience that eating should be.

Gently satisfy your appetite. Eat with awareness and attention to your physical appetite, so that you eat when you are hungry and stop when you are comfortably satisfied but not overfull.

We believe that the enjoyment of a meal is not necessarily dependent on quantity. Start by serving yourself smaller portions than you are used to, and decide if you are still hungry before you eat more. Work on distinguishing between physical hunger and other reasons for eating, such as dealing with stress, anxiety, or boredom, or fulfilling other emotional needs.

These decisions are important, because eating too much is bad not only for the body but for the brain. Recent studies have shown that a diet too high in calories can increase your risk of memory loss and premature brain aging. There's also a definite relationship between exceeding a healthy weight as measured by your body mass index (BMI) and cognitive decline. In a 2011 study released by the Mayo Clinic in Scottsdale, Arizona, older people who consumed more than two thousand calories a day had more than double the risk of memory loss compared with those who ate fewer than fifteen hundred calories a day.

Establish a pattern of eating regularly. You're more likely to be satisfied with reasonable portions if you don't let yourself become ravenously hungry between meals. Plan to eat every three to four hours, basing your eating on a pattern of breakfast, lunch, and dinner, with an afternoon snack—especially if there is a long time between lunch and dinner. It's easy to forget to eat when you are very busy, but regular meals may help you maintain your energy level throughout the day and decrease the potential of overeating in the evening.

What's more, the brain runs on *glucose,* the simplest form of sugar. One of the best things you can do to support brain health is to manage blood sugar by feeding your brain throughout the day with small, frequent meals. Each of these meals should be composed of complex carbohydrates, such as whole grains, vegetables, fruits, beans, and nuts and seeds, along with a healthy lean protein and a moderate amount of fat. This combination is the optimal way to deliver a sustained breakdown of glucose to the brain. The brain receives the glucose from the carbs right away. Later, once the proteins are broken down, it will receive those nutrients as glucose, and then much later, it can tap into glucose that has been stored in the richest, most concentrated way, via fat. So when you eat five times a day instead of one or two giant, calorie-laden meals, you are helping to create and deliver a constant supply of glucose that keeps the brain strong.

Another benefit of switching to this type of eating pattern is that many people see an improvement in their mood because their brain is receiving a steady supply of fuel. The brain doesn't like the ups and downs and highs and lows of erratic eating, or starvation, causing some to feel emotional or irritable when they are dieting and not taking in enough calories, or spreading meals too far apart during the day.

The Importance of Creating a Memorable Meal

It's not just what you eat; it's also *how* you eat that can help improve your mind and mood. The memory of a meal is just as important as its nutritional value in terms of brain health. Your memories are what prompt you to search out more similar experiences in order to create more positive memories. So the momentary pleasure and nutrition that you get from food are just as important as the pleasurable experience that stays with you.

For example, if I told you I was giving you a glass of fabulously expensive wine, even though it might really be the $9.99 store special, I can guarantee you would remember the whole meal as being exceptional. In this case, it's the expectation set up by previous memories of drinking good wine that forces your brain to create an extraordinary experience in real time, even though you are drinking ordinary wine.

What's more, the way you eat and the order in which you eat makes a big difference in how you remember a meal. Research has shown us that the end of a meal is particularly important for creating positive memories. That's why we traditionally end important meals, like dinner, with a dessert that is sweet and rich—both sweetness and richness are satisfying to the brain.

At Canyon Ranch we strive to craft perfect meals that are meant to enhance your ability to enjoy and remember a great meal. We pace out meals slowly, starting with an appetizer, usually a soup or salad, followed by a main course, and finally a small serving of dessert. This is designed to enhance the memory of the meal, so that when you get home you can re-create this ritual of eating and produce more of your own positive memories associated with food.

Start with the Basics of Good Nutrition

Over the next month you'll learn why you need certain foods to achieve the best brain health. Each week you'll add another component of better eating to your routine, ramping up good habits and trading old, unhealthy patterns for new, better suggestions. Our mission is to inspire you to make a commitment to healthy living through healthy eating. By following this program, you'll begin to see real changes in the way you think as well as the way you look and feel.

At Canyon Ranch, we promote the basic tenets of what many call a Mediterranean diet. This includes a wide variety of whole foods: vegetables, fruits, beans, nuts/seeds, whole grains, and fish and lean proteins in their most natural, unprocessed forms. The following suggestions are the backbone of this type of eating plan.

Smaller Portions of Lean Proteins

Foods that are high in protein are packed with nutrients that support brain health. The neurotransmitters, or chemical messengers sent from the brain, are mostly made of amino acids, the building blocks of protein. Raising the levels of specific amino acids, such as tyrosine, causes neurons to manufacture norepinephrine and dopamine, two neurotransmitters that promote alertness and activity. That may be why many people feel more alert through the afternoon after they have eaten a protein-rich lunch.

Including protein with every meal will also help stabilize your energy levels throughout the day. These types of meals fill you up so that you will feel satisfied and not hungry. Our favorite sources of protein are fish, poultry, and plant-based proteins such as beans and soy foods, but there are many other plant and animal foods that can satisfy your protein needs, such as grass-fed lean meats. Don't overlook nut butters, low-fat or nonfat yogurt and cheeses, and eggs.

While it's important to eat protein at every meal, it's equally important to keep these portions small. Most Americans eat far more protein than they need, and this habit leads us to consume too much saturated fat. A moderate serving size is twenty to forty grams of protein at every meal, which is about three to six ounces of animal protein. Think of the perfect serving as approximately the size of the palm of your hand. You can also avoid consuming extra fats by choosing skinless chicken breasts and lean or well-trimmed cuts of grass-fed red meats, such as loin and round, with less visible marbling.

Most of us can easily add protein choices to lunch or dinner. However, it turns out that the traditional American breakfast of toast or cereal with a splash of milk is a good place to make a change that can enhance your cognitive performance. One 2002 study from the Swiss Federal Institute of Technology showed that without protein as part of breakfast, cognitive function declined, but when participants ate a breakfast higher in protein, their mental acuity increased due to the shift in neurotransmitter production. By including eggs, nut butters, or other protein-rich foods in your morning routine, you will have increased sharpness and mental focus to start your day off right. Low-fat yogurt is filling, high in protein—especially Greek-style varieties—and high in calcium. In a 2011 Harvard study, yogurt was found to be one of only two foods directly linked to long-term weight loss. A second study, published in the *American Journal of Clinical Nutrition,* also links dairy products to decreasing oxidative and inflammatory stress, especially for those with metabolic syndrome.

Good sources of protein include:

Beans
Chicken or turkey, skinless
Eggs
Grass-fed lean meat (loin/round cuts)
Low-fat dairy products, including milk, cheese, and yogurt
Nuts/seeds
Protein powder
Soy: edamame, tofu, tempeh, soy nuts
Wild fish

Whole Grains

Whole-grain foods are made from wheat, rice, oats, cornmeal, barley, or another cereal grain. Bread, pasta, oatmeal, breakfast cereals, tortillas, and grits are examples of grain products. Whole grains contain the entire grain kernel—the bran, germ, and endosperm. This is critical because the bran, or outer layer of the grain, is where the fiber resides and is why whole-grain choices are nutritionally better for you as compared with *refined* grains, those that have been stripped of the outer layer. In addition, the inner grain—the germ—provides many important nutrients, such as vitamin E, the B complex vitamins, fiber, and minerals. Whole grains provide an abundance of antioxidants, as well as other vitamins and minerals—the nutrients the body needs to work properly—and are therefore critical for good health. The fiber content of whole grains slows the rate of glucose absorption from the stomach and helps stabilize blood sugar levels for several hours after eating, providing energy and appetite control.

Making the switch to whole grains is critical for improving brain health because many people who are experiencing cognitive dysfunction may be deficient in B vitamins, a nutrient group that is common in whole grains. An average of 66 percent of B vitamins that naturally occur in whole grains are removed in the process of creating white flour. Worse still, the calorie content of refined white flour is actually about 10 percent higher than that of whole-grain flour because of everything that has been taken out.

The following chart can help you transition toward whole grains. Focus on the "Foods to Choose" as you minimize the "Foods to Avoid." One easy way to begin is by purchasing whole wheat or whole-grain versions of your favorite breads, cereals, crackers, pasta, pitas, sandwich buns and rolls, pretzels, and tortillas. Look at the ingredient list to make sure the first ingredient begins with the word *whole,* as in *whole wheat* or *whole rye.* One exception is rolled or steel-cut oats, which are also considered to be whole grains.

These healthier options are available in most supermarkets. You can even make good whole-grain choices, like brown rice or whole wheat pizza, at many of your favorite restaurants.

Foods to Choose: Whole Grains	Foods to Avoid: Refined Grains
Amaranth	Barley (pearled)
Barley (unhulled)	Corn bread
Brown rice	Corn or white-flour tortillas
Buckwheat	Couscous
Bulgur (cracked wheat)	Grits
Millet	Cornflakes breakfast cereals
Muesli	White rice
Oats (rolled and steel cut)	Instant oatmeal
Popcorn (air popped)	Traditional pastas
Quinoa	
Sorghum	
Whole wheat or whole-grain pasta	
Whole-grain cornmeal	
Whole rye	
Whole-grain breakfast cereals	
Wild rice	

Fill Your Plate with Colorful Vegetables and Fruits

Eat eight to ten servings of vegetables and fruit daily. A typical portion of either is half a cup, or the size of a medium apple or orange (about the size of a baseball).

Fruits and vegetables are nutrient-rich foods filled with fiber, antioxidants, vitamins, and minerals. One important study from Tufts University's Jean Mayer USDA Human Nutrition Research Center on Aging reported the positive effects of wild blueberries on mild cognitive impairment. And according to a 2006 study from Rush University Medical Center, just 2.8 servings (about a cup and a half) of blueberries a day have been shown to decrease memory loss.

The brain-protective properties of fruits and vegetables are found in their flavonoids: the compounds that give plants their color. These flavonoids act as powerful antioxidants. Studies have shown that people who eat fruits and vegetables in accordance with the Canyon Ranch recommendations outlined here—which are consistent with the U.S. Dietary Guidelines—are associated with a lower risk of several diseases, including cognitive decline. What's more, a study from the *American Journal of Epidemiology* noted that a diet high in flavonoids is associated with less memory loss over a ten-year period.

Each day, try to eat all the colors of the rainbow: greens that are rich in antioxidants, such as lutein and zeaxanthin, as well as trace minerals and B vitamins; reds like watermelon and tomatoes that are rich in lycopene; oranges, such as squash and sweet potatoes, that are rich in carotenoids; and blues and purples, including blueberries and grapes, that are rich in flavonoids called anthocyanins. Other colors to consider are browns, such as nuts, tea, whole grains, black olives, beans, and coffee, which are highly concentrated in important nutrient compounds.

Consider adding fruit to your breakfast and eating a large salad once a day, a vegetable or fruit combined with protein for an afternoon snack, and a generous portion of vegetables at lunch and dinner. Whenever possible, choose fresh, organic, locally grown vegetables and fruits that are in season. Frozen options are a possibility as well. The term *organic* signifies food products that are manufactured, grown, or raised under the authority of the Organic Foods Production Act (OFPA). Organic farmers avoid hormones, antibiotics, and genetic modifications and use minimal fungicides and pesticides and non-farm-produced fertilizers. Consequently, fewer pollutants will make their way onto your dinner table and into your body and your brain. While eating organic will not "boost the brain," it will help lower your body burden, as we discussed in chapter 4.

Making the Best Organic Choices

The USDA organic designation can apply to fruits and vegetables, meats and poultry, dairy, grains, and even processed and packaged foods. With so many options, it's sometimes hard to choose where to start. The Environmental Working Group's website (www.ewg.org) has a terrific Shopper's Guide to Pesticides in Produce, which lists the fruits and vegetables that have the most, and the least, amount of pesticide residue. You can use this list to make an informed decision about when to buy organic.

Limit Sugar and Avoid Artificial Sweeteners

Savor the natural sweetness of whole foods such as fresh fruits, vegetables, and nuts, and limit your consumption of foods high in added sugar as well as artificial sweeteners. It is tempting to replace sugar with artificial sweeteners, but there are potential health risks associated with them, and by consuming them frequently you are activating further cravings for sweets. Be aware of artificial sweeteners hidden in cereals, yogurts, diet beverages, and other prepared foods.

If you must sweeten, use small amounts of pure maple syrup, honey, brown rice syrup, blackstrap molasses, or natural sugar. Choose fruit for dessert, and stir fresh fruit or all-fruit preserves into plain yogurt for a quick breakfast or snack.

Choose Healthy Fats

Fat is an essential part of a healthy diet, but the type of fat you consume is just as important to your health as is the amount. There are two types of fat: *saturated*, which is typically solid at room temperature; and *unsaturated*—including both polyunsaturated and monounsaturated—which is plant-based and is typically liquid at room temperature. The healthiest choices for your brain are the *monounsaturated fats* found in extra virgin olive oil, canola oil, avocado, olives, and nuts. Easy ways to get these good fats into your diet include making your own salad dressing using an organic, cold-pressed olive oil; sautéing vegetables in olive oil and garlic instead of margarine or butter; eating a small handful of nuts each day; and adding avocado slices to sandwiches and salads.

Another healthy source of plant-based fats is *polyunsaturated fatty acids* (PUFAs) found in most vegetable, nut, and seed oils, as well as fish. PUFAs are a rich source of essential fatty acids that are critical for brain function. These are also associated with improving cholesterol ratios and reducing the risk of cardiovascular disease.

Saturated fats raise the levels of total blood cholesterol and "bad" LDL cholesterol, which can increase your risk of cardiovascular disease. To reduce your intake of saturated fat, consume low-fat dairy products (preferably organic), such as milk and yogurt, and choose lower-fat cheeses that are harder and drier, such as feta, Parmesan, and part-skim mozzarella. Limit your consumption of foods made with butter and cream. Experiment with substitutes for full-fat dairy products in recipes, such as evaporated skim milk. Use the lowest appropriate heating temperatures for the shortest length of time when you are using cooking oils to avoid overexposure to high heat, which can cause unhealthy chemical changes in these types of foods.

Last, avoid any packaged goods with the words *trans fat* or *hydrogenated oils* in the ingredients list. Trans fats raise "bad" LDL and lower "good" HDL cholesterol in addition to triggering inflammation in the body. Many fast foods—especially those that are fried—are loaded with trans fats, although restaurants are getting better at removing them, and in some parts of the country, they have been banned altogether.

One important brain nutrient that comes from fat is *choline,* a precursor to the neurotransmitter acetylcholine. Choline is an important nutrient for improving cognitive function. According to a 2011 study, people who get plenty of choline in their diets may perform better on memory tests and be less likely to show brain changes associated with dementia. Choline is found in abundance in egg yolks. Eggs are a perfect protein because they can be cooked with little or no added fat. For years we were told to eat the whites of eggs and throw out the yolks because yolks were thought to be high in cholesterol. However, we now know two important facts about egg yolks: First, you're throwing out a nutrient-rich portion. And contrary to popular opinion, consumption of eggs won't necessarily increase cholesterol for the majority of people. In fact, the yolks contain health-promoting antioxidants such as lutein and important minerals such as iron. So don't throw out the good stuff, and enjoy eggs on a regular basis.

BE A FOOD DETECTIVE

We know it is a confusing nutrition world out there. Many "low fat" processed foods seem to be tempting options, but they are often loaded with sodium, corn syrup, and other sweeteners and may still be too high in fat to actually be good for you. Foods labeled "trans fat free" can still contain up to a full gram of these harmful fats per serving. And while "multigrain" sounds promising, it's often not much better for you than standard white bread, because the mix between whole grains and refined grains may not be in your favor.

The next time you're in the supermarket, become a food detective and read labels carefully! The USDA has standardized food labels, making the information more accessible than ever. The information in the top section contains product-specific content, including serving size and calories per serving. The middle section provides nutrition facts: the nutrient breakdown of each serving, comparing it with the Daily

Values (for 2,000- and 2,500-calorie diets) the government recommends. This provides suggested dietary information for important nutrients, including fats, sodium, and fiber; can help you decide whether a food is high or low in a certain nutrient; and can be used to compare one product with another.

Serving sizes have also been standardized to make it easier to compare similar foods, and are provided in familiar units such as cups or pieces. The size of the serving on the food package influences the number of calories and all the nutrient amounts listed on the top part of the label. Pay attention to the recommended serving size, and especially the estimation of how many servings there are in the food package, before you start eating. You may be surprised to learn that you are eating many more calories than you think. This is especially true of foods sold in large packages, such as potato chips or cookies. Calories are important to monitor because they let you know how much cellular energy you get from a single serving of a particular food. Many Americans consume more calories than they need, and at the same time are taking in fewer nutrients. When you consume too many calories for your body to process, the remainder becomes stored as body fat.

While the Nutrition Facts panel found on packaged goods is important, the ingredient list is the key to clean eating. We encourage you to choose items made with predominantly whole-food ingredients. The ingredients are listed by volume, in descending order. Therefore, the first few ingredients are most important. And while you're at it, shop at the perimeter of the

Talk to Your Doctor

Talk to your doctors about these suggestions for changing your eating routine. They will be glad to know you are taking proactive steps to improve your brain health. They will also be able to monitor if any of the nutrients or foods suggested here are interfering with your current health regimen. For example, while grapefruit is a significant source of vitamin C and antioxidants, it isn't a great choice for those taking certain medications, such as statins to lower cholesterol, because it can increase the amount of drugs circulating in the bloodstream.

store first; this will naturally limit the packaged/processed foods you purchase.

30 Days of Neuro-Nutrition

Beyond the basics of good nutrition, following this plan improves brain health because it emphasizes specific foods that enhance your brain function. We call this *neuro-nutrition*. Over the next four weeks, you'll learn how to make small but lasting changes. You'll also see that many of the foods that are good for one area of health also improve others. This is one of the most exciting findings in nutritional science: eating better improves all areas of health, literally head to toe.

For example, the brain and all of its individual neurons are made of fat and the essential fatty acids that we must obtain through diet. These neurons then communicate with one another via chemical messengers (neurotransmitters) between them, as well as hormones and enzymes that cause chemical changes and control all body processes.

You'll also learn about specific types of foods that help lower your risk of or reverse symptoms associated with many of the diseases linked to declining brain health, including inflammation, oxidative stress, heart disease, and diabetes.

Week One Focus: Lowering Inflammation

As you learned in chapter 2, inflammation is the healing response that occurs when there is an injury or infection. However, too much inflammation in effect clogs up the brain and can contribute to mild cognitive impairment, and ultimately dementia. And when inflammation affects the body, its related illnesses affect the brain.

Genetics may predispose you to increased or systemic inflammation, yet lifestyle also has a strong influence on the process. The foods we eat have a tremendous impact on the level of inflammation in the

body, and the typical Western high-carbohydrate, high-fat diet contributes significantly. According to the University of Maryland Medical
Center, the typical American diet alone causes inflammation.

Luckily, you can choose other foods that can help lower inflammation throughout the body and the brain, beginning at the cellular
level. Every cell membrane contains—and requires—fatty acids in
order to survive. However, neither the brain nor the body produces
these essential fatty acids: they must come from the diet. The most
prominent is a long-chain omega-6 fatty acid called *arachidonic acid*
(AA). This particular acid chain is produced after the consumption
of *linoleic acid,* found primarily in animal fats, vegetable oils, and
the foods prepared with these fats. Long-chain omega-3 fatty acids
are also found in cell membranes and must also be consumed in
food. The most prominent omega-3 fatty acid is *eicosapentaenoic acid*
(EPA), which is produced from the consumption of *alpha-linolenic
acid* found in flaxseed or flax oil, walnuts, and soy foods. EPA is
also available directly from fatty fish, grass-fed animal meats, and
omega-3-enriched eggs.

EPAs have been shown to have a positive effect on the brain, alleviating or diminishing depression and increasing executive function.
In one 2011 study from Oregon Health & Science University, healthy
seniors whose diets contained higher levels of omega-3 fatty acids
performed better on certain measures of thinking abilities, and also
tended to have larger brain volume. At the same time, seniors who ate
high levels of trans fats had more brain shrinkage than those with lower
levels of these unhealthy fats.

Another omega-3 fatty acid is *docosahexaenoic acid* (DHA), which
is found in cold-water fatty fish, such as salmon, and omega-3-enriched
eggs and is also formed from EPA. Your body needs DHA for proper
brain functioning. It is involved in the earliest stages of brain development as well as visual function, and can continue to enhance brain
health throughout your life.

All of these fatty acids are released from cell membranes each time
a cell receives a signal to respond to a biological need. They are then
transformed into substances that influence inflammation throughout

the brain and the body. The substances produced from AA may increase levels of inflammation, while those produced by EPA and DHA are anti-inflammatory, decreasing these levels. An abundance of EPA in cell membranes can further reduce inflammation by providing more competition in the reactions that typically use AA.

Week One Goal: Choose Anti-Inflammatory Foods

In order to lower inflammation, you need to focus on foods that are known to decrease it, those that are high in the "healthy fats" called essential fatty acids. The typical Western diet provides an excess of omega-6 fatty acids compared with lower levels of omega-3 fatty acids. The optimal level of omega-3 intake is three to five grams per day. In order to achieve this, we at Canyon Ranch recommend at least two servings a week of fish rich in EPA, and one source of omega-3 fatty acids every day.

This week you will maximize the anti-inflammatory potential of your diet every day by:

1. Choosing foods high in EPA from the lists below.

2. Minimizing AA intake. The largest source of AA is the visible fat of meat, but all meats, poultry, shellfish, and egg yolks contain this fatty acid. We recommend trimming all fat from meat and eating smaller servings of these foods less often. By choosing omega-3-enriched eggs, you are getting a better balance of healthy fats.

3. Aim for a healthy blend of omega-6-rich fatty acids (such as linoleic acid, found in most vegetable oils) with foods high in EPA. Focus on using cold-pressed, preferably organic oils and balance your intake of omega-6 oils, including corn, safflower, soybean, or sunflower oils, with omega-

3-rich, cold-pressed canola or extra virgin olive oil when cooking and baking and in salad dressings. Keep your cooking oils in the refrigerator, as they can easily become rancid. You could keep a small glass bottle of olive or canola oil in your pantry while the bulk is stored in the fridge. Never store oils near the stove or oven, as they can be affected by heat.

The Best Food Sources of Omega-3 Fatty Acids

Anchovies

Chia seeds

Chunk light canned tuna (skipjack)

Dark green leafy vegetables

Flaxseed and flaxseed oil

Hemp seed and hemp seed oil

Herring

Lake trout

Mackerel

Omega-3-enriched eggs

Pumpkin seeds

Salmon

Sardines

Soy

Tuna (fresh)

Walnuts

Anti-Inflammatory-Rich Foods

Many other types of foods are also considered to be anti-inflammatory; for example, spices like ginger and turmeric are effective anti-inflammatories when they are used liberally. Fresh foods in this category include:

Apples

Bell peppers

Dark berries

Grapes

Kohlrabi

Onions

Pears

Sour cherries

Some foods contain *salicylates,* the active ingredient in aspirin. These foods have been traditionally used as natural pain relievers because they lower inflammation, just as aspirin does. These should all be included in your diet this week—unless you are sensitive to aspirin, as salicylate is an aspirinlike substance that can cause adverse reactions, including asthma and hives.

Black pepper	Pickles
Cinnamon	Prunes
Curry	Raisins
Dill	Raspberries
Fenugreek	Rosemary
Honey	Sage
Licorice	Tarragon
Mint (fresh)	Thyme
Mustard	Turmeric
Oregano	Worcestershire sauce
Paprika	

THE HEALTHIEST FISH OPTIONS

Eating fish is definitely one of the best ways to get more omega-3 in your diet. However, not all fish are equally good choices. Unfortunately, the damage we've done to our environment, and the way that some fish are farmed and raised, makes some choices better than others. Yet it's important to keep in mind that while there are legitimate concerns regarding potential contaminants and environmental issues, experts agree that the benefits of eating a variety of fish far outweigh any risks.

All types of tuna are excellent sources of omega-3s, but because it is such a large fish, it is significantly affected by pollutants, especially mercury. This heavy metal tends to *bioaccumulate,* which means that large fish like tuna store mercury in their liver and body fat, making frequent consumption hazardous to your brain and body; as you've learned, mercury toxicity can result in memory loss, tremors, and increased risk for certain types of cancers.

Other fish may also contain contaminants. Potentially dangerous compounds found in fish include chemical pollutants from agricultural runoff: pesticides sprayed in the air find their way into the water supply and then accumulate in the fatty tissue of fish. Fish that are lower on the food chain or are plant eaters typically contain fewer toxins, while predatory fish such as shark, swordfish, and king mackerel contain higher levels.

Enjoy these fish and shellfish frequently, as they have the lowest contaminant levels:

Anchovies	Mussel (blue)
Butterfish	Oysters
Catfish	Perch (ocean)
Clams	Pollack
Cod	Salmon (canned)
Crab	Salmon (Alaskan)
Crawfish	Sardines
Croaker (Atlantic)	Scallops
Flatfish	Shad (American)
Flounder	Shrimp
Haddock	Sole
Hake	Squid
Herring	Tilapia
Jacksmelt	Trout (freshwater)
Mackerel (Atlantic)	Tuna (canned)
Mackerel (chub)	Whitefish
Mahimahi	Whiting
Mullet	

Limit these fish to six ounces—one serving—per month, due to their moderate levels:

Bass (saltwater, black, striped)
Bluefish
Buffalo fish
Carp
Chilean sea bass
Croaker (white)
Grouper
Halibut
Lobster (Northern American)
Mackerel (Spanish)
Marlin
Monkfish
Orange roughy

Perch (freshwater)
Sablefish
Scorpion fish
Sea trout
Sheepshead
Skate
Snapper
Tilefish (Atlantic)
Tuna (bigeye)
Tuna (canned, albacore)
Tuna (skipjack)
Tuna (yellowfin)

Avoid the following fish and shellfish because of their potentially high mercury content:

King mackerel
Shark
Swordfish
Tilefish (from the Gulf of Mexico)
Tuna (bluefin)

Sustainability

You can also choose your fish by how it is caught or raised. The best choices are those fish that are abundant and caught or farmed in environmentally safe ways. For example, salmon is a good fatty fish choice if it is wild caught. Farmed salmon has been clouded with a myriad of questionable practices, the most important of which is that we are not always told what farm-raised fish have been fed. Some are fed cornmeal, while others are fed ground-up fish. Beta-carotene is often added to enhance the color of farm-raised fish. Farmed salmon tends to be higher in PCB levels than wild salmon. Last, farm-raised fish are often given antibiotics, which you then consume when you eat the fish.

Here are some guidelines for selecting salmon:

- Wild Alaskan salmon has been shown to have the least contamination. Wild salmon from Washington State and British Columbia are the best choices.
- Canned salmon is usually wild Alaskan salmon.
- Select organic farm raised if available.
- Farmed salmon from Washington State and Chile have the lowest contaminant levels in the farmed category.

The following is a list of other sustainable fish choices:

Catfish	Mahimahi
Caviar (sturgeon)	Mussels
Clams	Oysters
Cod	Pollack (wild caught from
Crab (Dungeness, Canada	Alaska)
snow, stone)	Striped bass
Halibut (Pacific)	Sturgeon bass
Herring (Atlantic/sardines)	Tilapia
Lobster (spiny U.S.)	Trout (rainbow)

WEEK TWO FOCUS: REDUCE OXIDATIVE STRESS

The best way to combat oxidative stress and free radicals is by first eating less and focusing on a diet rich in antioxidants: any substances that prevent or reduce oxidative stress. These foods neutralize free radicals by donating an electron to make the molecule stable; the stability helps prevent cellular damage.

The best sources of antioxidants are the healthiest food choices:

vegetables, fruit, tea and coffee, nuts, seeds, and whole grains. A diet rich in antioxidants has also been clinically shown to delay the earliest symptoms of Alzheimer's disease. Researchers at the Institute of Biochemistry and Molecular Biology I of the Heinrich Heine University in Düsseldorf, Germany, investigated the relationship between antioxidant status and cognitive performance. Their results indicated that people of any age with a high daily intake of fruits and vegetables have higher antioxidant levels, lower levels of oxidative stress, and better cognitive performance than healthy subjects of any age consuming low amounts of fruits and vegetables.

Getting your antioxidants directly from food sources appears to be a better choice than taking supplements of the same nutrients. Natural foods contain an unmatchable combination of beneficial substances. Each food can contain thousands of different antioxidants, and in many cases it's not known which of these substances provide health benefits, whereas a supplement typically contains a single type of antioxidant. In addition to their antioxidant content, antioxidant-rich foods are also high in fiber, protein, and other vitamins and minerals and are typically low in saturated fat and cholesterol. This means that not only are they good for combating free radicals; they are crucial for your overall good health, and particularly for that of the brain.

WEEK TWO GOAL: EAT MORE VEGGIES AND FRUITS

The goal for this week is to make antioxidants available at every meal. You can make a major improvement in your diet by finding at least three new ways to add vegetables and fruit to your daily routine. Consider adding fruit to your breakfast, enjoy a medium-to-large salad once a day, and be sure that each meal includes vegetables and/or fruit. Always include fruit or vegetables in your afternoon snack. This is probably the easiest way to add fruit and vegetables to your diet and, at the same time, break bad habits of choosing foods with higher fat content or simple carbs as a way to fill you up between meals.

The Best Antioxidant Choices

There are thousands of different antioxidants, and each performs varying functions. Their beneficial value is almost always in the plant's pigments—their color—including the bark, rinds, seeds, leaves, fruits, and flowers. One good rule of thumb is, the darker the color, the higher the antioxidant value. Wash your fruits and veggies thoroughly, because you'll want to eat the skins in order to reap the most benefits.

The following chart shows many of the antioxidants that scientists have identified as having significant nutritional benefits:

Antioxidant	Found In
Alpha-linolenic acid	Flaxseed, soy, walnuts
Alpha-lipoic acid	Broccoli, spinach and other greens, potatoes, red meat
Anthocyanins	Red or purple grapes, red apples, red bell peppers, berries, red cabbage, cherries, eggplant, plums, red pears, red wine
Astaxanthin	Salmon
Carotenoids: carotenes	Green, orange, and yellow fruits and vegetables, including kale, mangoes, oranges, collard greens, cantaloupe, peaches, apricots, carrots, spinach, sweet potatoes, Swiss chard, pumpkin, red and yellow peppers, corn, papaya, tangerines
Capsaicin	Chili peppers
Lycopene	Tomatoes, tomato products (ketchup, pasta sauce), red grapefruit, guava, dried apricots, watermelon
Curcumin	Turmeric, curry, cumin
Monoterpene, limonene	Citrus (peel, membrane), mint, caraway, thyme, coriander
Quercetin	Pear skin, apple skin, bell pepper, kohlrabi, tomato leaves, onion, wine, grape juice
Resveratrol	Chocolate, wine, grapes
Ubiquinone	Mackerel, sardines, beef, peanuts, spinach

Antioxidant	Found In
Vitamin C (ascorbic acid)	Citrus fruits, green peppers, broccoli, green leafy vegetables, black currants, strawberries, blueberries, raw cabbage tomatoes
Vitamin E	Asparagus, olives, wheat germ, nuts, seeds, soy, whole grains, green leafy vegetables, kiwifruit, vegetable oil, fish-liver oil

Vegetables

Colorful vegetables are rich in antioxidants. Eat a wide variety of vegetables every day, and enjoy them raw, steamed, grilled, sautéed, or stir-fried with your favorite seasonings. Some of the best choices are:

Artichokes	Collard greens
Arugula	Daikon
Asparagus	Kale
Avocados	Kohlrabi
Beets	Mizuna
Bok choy	Radish
Broccoli	Rutabaga
Broccoli rabe	Spinach
Brussels sprouts	Tomato
Cabbage	Turnip
Cauliflower	Watercress

Fruits

While all fruits have antioxidants, some have more than others. Choose from this list whenever possible, especially when they are locally grown, organic, and in season:

Apples	Blackberries
Black currants	Blueberries

Cherries
Cranberries
Figs
Guava
Mango

Oranges
Plums
Pomegranate
Raspberries
Strawberries

Soup Satisfies

Starting meals with a fruit soup or vegetable soup takes the edge off your appetite and is another effective way to add antioxidants to your day. Choose highly colored soups with a base of low-fat yogurt or vegetable stock instead of cream. Pureed vegetables, like squash, make for very satisfying soups.

Spices and Herbs

Another easy and efficient way to add antioxidants to your diet is by flavoring your meals. Spices do not add a single calorie to food preparation. Cayenne is thought to act as an anti-inflammatory and antioxidant. Cinnamon has antibacterial and anti-inflammatory properties, and it also has been shown to have a positive effect on insulin sensitivity. Turmeric and ginger are most noted for their anti-inflammatory properties, reducing pain and swelling in people with arthritis. Turmeric (curcumin) may decrease the formation of amyloid protein deposits in the brain, characteristic in people with Alzheimer's disease.

Don't be shy when you are cooking with spices: you'll need to use a tablespoon or more to make a significant impact. The ones that are highest in antioxidants are:

Cardamom
Chili powder
Cinnamon
Clove
Coriander
Cumin
Curry powder
Garlic

Ginger
Mustard seed
Paprika
Parsley
Pepper (black, white, cayenne—any type of pepper)
Turmeric

Herbs are often available both fresh and dried. The fresh ones have the highest antioxidant values. If fresh are not available, use the dried version in one-third the amount called for with fresh. The following herbs are the most potent antioxidants:

Basil	Sage
Dill	Savory
Marjoram	Tarragon
Oregano	Thyme
Peppermint	

Enjoy Your Coffee

Coffee is the most common way Americans get their antioxidants. Coffee has been shown to reduce the risk of Alzheimer's, Parkinson's disease, diabetes, heart disease, gallstones, and kidney stones. Be aware that caffeine increases urinary loss of calcium; this loss can weaken bones, unless you put milk in your coffee, providing calcium to offset this effect.

Coffee's high concentration of caffeine has been shown to enhance neuronal activity, and it may improve short-term memory. The way that you brew your coffee also makes a difference in terms of keeping it free from unnecessary chemicals. The safest way to brew coffee is by brewing it through a brown-paper filter. White-paper filters are bleached, so they will have remnants of dioxins and traces of even banned substances like PCBs. Paper filters also remove the one dangerous compound in coffee, called cafestol. This compound has been shown to raise cholesterol, by up to forty or fifty points in some people. The types of coffee brewing that do not remove cafestol include cappuccino, espresso, a French press, percolated coffee, and the single-cup pod dispensers, because they don't use paper. So if you're using a brewing method that doesn't use paper, after you make your coffee, pour it through brown paper to remove the cafestol. A reasonable intake of caffeine is two to three (eight-ounce) cups of regular coffee per day, unless you find that it disrupts sleep, upsets your stomach, or causes a rapid heartbeat or anxiety.

Tea provides another caffeine option, but you have to drink a lot of it in order to match the medicinal effect of coffee. Teas, especially white and green tea, are very high in antioxidants and have a positive effect on cognitive function. Herbal teas are rich in antioxidants, but without the caffeine, they are not as effective in enhancing brain health.

Highly caffeinated sodas, including diet sodas, are not good choices for getting your caffeine buzz. Carbonated beverages of all stripes contain high levels of phosphates, which are bad for your teeth and bones because phosphates deplete calcium. They are particularly detrimental if you are over the age of forty, when the kidneys begin to become less efficient at processing phosphorous.

ANTIOXIDANT-RICH DESSERTS

When you do indulge, you might as well be taking care of your brain at the same time. You can choose any combination of dark chocolate, fruit, and nuts for a sweet and satisfying dessert. The cocoa that is the basis for chocolate is packed with antioxidants. In one 2003 study comparing the chemical anticancer activity in beverages known to contain antioxidants, researchers from Cornell University found that cocoa has nearly twice the antioxidants of red wine and up to three times those found in green tea. Choose dark chocolate with the highest percentage of cocoa (a minimum of 70 percent).

Berries are naturally high in fiber and vitamin C, and many pack plenty of manganese, folate, and potassium. Dried, sweetened berries can be high in calories, but a cup of fresh berries contains only forty to eighty calories. That makes them a guilt-free part of your diet that delivers a powerhouse of nutrients and potential health benefits.

While many nuts are high in antioxidants, walnuts lead the pack. They have a combination of more healthful antioxidants and higher-quality antioxidants than any other nut. It takes only about seven walnuts a day to get the potential health benefits. Walnuts also contain a number of potentially neuroprotective compounds, including vitamin E, folate, melatonin, and omega-3 fatty acids. The heat required in roasting nuts generally reduces the quality of the antioxidants. However, walnuts are typically eaten raw, so you get the full effectiveness of the antioxidants.

Week Three Focus:
Master Blood-Sugar Regulation

Our bodies digest all types of carbohydrates into glucose to be used for energy in every cell. The delivery of glucose to the cells is facilitated by the hormone insulin. Insulin is produced by specialized cells in the pancreas and released into the bloodstream after food is eaten or when glucose produced by the liver enters circulation. Although carbohydrates trigger the largest insulin release, both protein and fat also cause a rise in insulin levels.

Insulin changes the permeability of cell membranes and allows glucose and other fuels to enter the cell. When these substances enter the cell, their levels in the blood are lowered. Normally this is a fine-tuned process providing a steady supply of glucose to the cell. When insulin receptors are not as responsive, glucose delivered to the cell is compromised, a condition known as insulin resistance. In response to this, the pancreas secretes even larger amounts of insulin. In the early stages of insulin resistance, blood glucose levels may be normal, but insulin levels are high. In some people, the pancreas eventually cannot meet the demand for insulin and serum glucose levels remain high, leading to diabetes.

Blood glucose levels are dynamic and fluctuate throughout the day and night in response to meals, physical activity, stress levels, hormone levels, and even circadian rhythms. They often affect how we feel, how much energy we have, and how clearly we think. Managing blood glucose is then an effective therapeutic strategy for controlling hunger, food cravings, energy and stress levels, and mood swings and improving brain function.

An added benefit of steady blood glucose levels is more stable insulin levels. Elevated insulin levels are related to high blood pressure, high cholesterol levels, hormonal imbalances, decreased immunity, increased inflammation, and an increased risk of heart disease. What's more, the highest production of insulin is found in the hippocampus, the region associated with memory, learning, and other cognitive functions. Insulin is also created in the hypothalamus, another area of the brain that regulates emotions and involuntary functions. The latest brain research links both diabetes and dementia to the brain chemical acetylcholine. A 2005 study from Brown University's Alpert Medical School, and a more recent 2008 study out of Sweden, found that insulin production in the brain declines as Alzheimer's disease advances. The Brown study showed that many features of Alzheimer's, such as cell death and development of plaque in the brain, appear to be linked to abnormalities in insulin signaling and glucose uptake. This finding is another reason some researchers believe that Alzheimer's disease and other vascular dementias could be referred to as type 3 diabetes.

THE GLYCEMIC INDEX AND GLYCEMIC LOAD

Foods vary greatly in their impact on blood sugar and insulin levels. The *glycemic index* (GI) is a rating given to carbohydrate-rich foods based on how much and how quickly they increase blood sugar. Lower glycemic carbohydrates such as whole unprocessed grains, legumes, and many fruits and vegetables digest slowly and raise blood sugar gradually. These foods do not result in large fluctuations in blood sugar, which may stimulate food cravings. In contrast, refined, processed carbohydrates raise blood sugar rapidly and lead to erratic blood-sugar patterns.

For More Information . . .

To see a complete listing of the glycemic index, visit the website www.glycemicindex.com.

A practical application of the glycemic index data is referred to as *glycemic load* (GL). This calculation reflects the total carbohydrates in a serving of food. For example, carrots are thought to be high in sugar. Yet the amount of carbohydrates in a typical serving of carrots is actually very small, giving it a low glycemic load. However, if you juiced an entire bunch of carrots, the glycemic load would be greater because of the increase in total carbohydrate content due to the larger portion consumed.

FILL UP WITH FIBER

The fiber found in whole grains and other sources is considered to be a supernutrient that not only controls insulin production but can help to regulate blood sugar and preserve cognitive function. A 2001 study from the University of Cardiff, in Wales, found that people with a higher fiber intake had less emotional distress, fewer cognitive difficulties, and less fatigue than their counterparts who consumed a smaller amount of fiber. The benefits of a high-fiber diet include the abundance of phytonutrients found in a plant-based diet, in addition to the positive impact on blood-sugar control.

This week, you'll begin to add more fiber to your diet. But don't take on too much too quickly. Possible side effects of a high-fiber diet include bloating, constipation, diarrhea, and intestinal gas. To minimize these uncomfortable side effects, plan to increase your fiber intake slowly over days or weeks, allowing the digestive system to adjust. Be sure to drink plenty of fluid, and avoid consuming dry fiber, such as bran or high-fiber cereal, without adequate fluids.

There are many types of dietary fibers that are typically grouped into one of two categories: soluble or insoluble. *Insoluble fiber* increases the bulk of waste material by absorbing water. Good sources of insoluble fiber include whole grains, legumes, fruits, and vegetables. *Soluble fiber* dissolves in water and can bind with sugars and fats, among other digestive waste products, increasing fecal excretion of these elements. This binding property slows or reduces the absorption of sugar and fats into the blood, thus helping to improve blood-sugar control and lower blood cholesterol.

Week 3 Goal:
Choose Foods That Help
Control Insulin Levels

The two most effective strategies that make cells more sensitive to insulin seem to be regular, vigorous exercise and weight loss if you are overweight. The foods you choose can help as well.

Make a point of trying a new whole-grain food every day this week, and continue to eat antioxidant-rich fruits and vegetables, which are typically high in fiber. On average, Americans consume fourteen grams or less of dietary fiber per day. The current recommended intake levels are significantly higher, so you'll need to try to get some fiber in every meal to reach these numbers:

ADULTS UNDER FIFTY YEARS:

Men: thirty-eight grams   Women: twenty-five grams

ADULTS OVER FIFTY YEARS:

Men: thirty grams   Women: twenty-one grams

At Canyon Ranch, one of our favorite fiber options is beans. The most colorful versions, such as lentils and red or black beans, contain powerful antioxidants. Beans are high in protein, low in fat, high in fiber, and low on the glycemic index, so they are a perfect choice. You can easily substitute them in any recipe that calls for ground beef, or add them to soups and salads. Try hummus

---

Quick Tips to Increase Fiber

- Eat the peel on vegetables and fruits (when possible)
- Add oat or wheat bran to cereal, casseroles, and lean ground meat
- Try a high-fiber cereal
- Try new or different whole grains
- Read labels carefully and choose the highest-fiber options whenever possible

(made from garbanzo beans/chickpeas) or other bean spreads, lentil and pea soups, and vegetarian chili.

Other good sources of fiber include:

Barley	Oat bran
Bran	Oatmeal
Brown rice	Quinoa
Bulgur	Sweet potatoes
Fruits	Wild rice
Legumes	

Choose Low-Glycemic Foods

The foods with the lowest glycemic index and glycemic load ratings are clearly the best choices in terms of carbohydrates. For this week, focus on the following foods and include them in your meals as often as possible:

Apples	Oranges
Apricots	Peaches
Beans (all varieties)	Peanuts
Carrots	Pears
Dark chocolate (greater than 70 percent cocoa)	Prunes
	Skim milk
Grapefruit	Soy milk
Grapes	Strawberries
Kiwi	Whole wheat bread
Low-fat yogurt	

Dietary Changes That Can
Help Control Blood Sugar

The following suggestions and strategies can work if you adopt them
as lifestyle changes:

- *Small, frequent meals:* Eating every three to four hours helps
  keep blood glucose and insulin levels low and stable.
- *Limit refined white flour and sugar:* Refined or processed
  grains and sugar rapidly raise blood glucose and insulin
  levels and are easy to eat in excess. Fructose, found in table
  sugar and high-fructose corn syrup, has been shown to make
  cells more insulin resistant.
- *Eat whole grains:* Whole grains seem to result in a lower
  insulin response.
- *Eat balanced meals:* Including a moderate portion of a
  protein-rich food and a moderate amount of healthy fat will
  help slow the absorption of carbohydrates.
- *Limit saturated fat:* Saturated fat intake is related to insulin
  resistance because it reduces the fluidity of cell membranes,
  decreasing receptor functioning.
- *Include omega-3 fatty acids:* These essential fatty acids may
  work to keep cell membranes fluid.
- *Use cinnamon liberally:* Cinnamon has been shown to
  improve glucose levels in individuals with diabetes and is
  thought to be helpful with insulin resistance.
- *Vitamin D:* Foods rich in this vitamin have been associated
  with maintaining insulin sensitivity in cell membranes
  and healthy functioning of the pancreas, where insulin is
  made. These include eggs, milk and dairy products, salmon,
  sardines, and tuna. A deficiency in vitamin D has also been
  linked to a higher risk of cognitive decline and Alzheimer's
  disease.

- *Chromium:* Foods rich in this trace mineral have a stabilizing effect on blood sugar. These include asparagus, black pepper, mushrooms, nuts, prunes, and raisins.
- *Magnesium:* Foods rich in this mineral have been shown to improve insulin sensitivity. These include almonds, blackstrap molasses, broccoli, lentils, millet, pumpkin seeds, spinach, sunflower seeds, tofu, and wheat germ.
- *Antioxidants:* A diet rich in antioxidants can help prevent the inflammation that often accompanies insulin resistance.

WEEK FOUR FOCUS: IMPROVE VASCULAR HEALTH

One important goal of improving brain performance is to keep the blood supply to the brain healthy. Your blood vessels must be able to deliver adequate oxygen and nutrients to the brain and throughout the body. If arterial plaque buildup reduces the blood flow to the brain, *ischemia,* or an inadequate blood supply, occurs, and brain function is impaired.

A second issue is maintaining healthy blood pressure, because abnormal pressure is a primary risk factor for stroke. Hypertension, or high blood pressure, occurs when elevated blood pressure intensifies inflammation, damaging blood vessels and increasing the potential for the buildup of plaque in vessels, which leads to a greater risk of heart attack and stroke. When plaque builds up in the arteries and blood flow is restricted, blood pressure further increases, making the heart work even harder.

We also know that poor vascular health affects the structure of the brain, leading to changes in cognition. In one longitudinal study from Wayne State University, researchers found that those suffering from hypertension had more white matter hyperintensities (WMH): dense regions of the brain that are more common with neurological disorders, psychiatric illnesses, or declines in intelligence. WMH progression is also correlated with declines in working memory. For this reason, we at Canyon Ranch believe that poor vascular health contributes to declines in cognition.

The Importance of B Vitamins

Another important aspect of vascular health is lowering levels of a particular amino acid known as *homocysteine*. Increased homocysteine levels are associated with a greater risk of heart disease. What's more, this compound is considered to be inflammatory, and its presence may indicate inadequate levels of several B vitamins. Many people with mild cognitive impairment are found to be deficient in various forms of vitamin B; this is why we strongly recommend increasing the intake of foods that are high in the B vitamins, such as folic acid and vitamins B_1, B_2, B_6, and B_{12}.

Increasing vitamin B_{12} may be crucial if you are following a vegetarian diet, which is naturally low in this vitamin. And as we get older, we may frequently lose the ability to absorb B_{12}. There are also a few medications that interfere with the absorption of B_{12}, specifically the acid blockers Prevacid, Prilosec, and Nexium and the diabetes drug Metformin.

Week Four Goal: Choose Foods That Promote Vascular Health

You can begin taking care of your heart and your vascular system through the foods you eat. A heart-healthy diet incorporates everything we've discussed in this chapter, beginning with following a Mediterranean diet. Researchers have known for a long time that a plant-based diet lowers the risk of heart disease and stroke. However, we now know that following a Mediterranean diet is also associated with fortifying small blood vessels in the brain and supports cognitive function. According to a 2012 study from the University of Miami, the primary component of the Mediterranean diet that was predictive of WMH volume was the ratio of monounsaturated to saturated fats. That's why choosing the best fats and avoiding the ones that are dangerous to the heart is so critical.

Embrace a DASH Diet

While medications to treat hypertension are available, research has shown that modest lifestyle and dietary changes can help treat and often delay or prevent high blood pressure. DASH stands for "dietary approaches to stop hypertension." This type of diet has been proven to lower blood pressure and is especially effective when paired with sodium restriction. A DASH diet is rich in vegetables, fruit, low-fat dairy products, and lean proteins and provides generous amounts of calcium, potassium, and magnesium.

Calcium is important because a low calcium intake may increase your risk of hypertension. Dairy products, fortified orange juice, fortified plant milks (soy, rice, almond), sesame seeds, bok choy, okra, almonds, tofu (fortified), and broccoli are all high in calcium.

Increasing potassium can help lower blood pressure. Potassium works with sodium to regulate the body's water balance. Research has shown that by increasing potassium and decreasing sodium, you can raise your likelihood of maintaining normal blood pressure. This mineral is found in tomatoes, potatoes, bananas, oranges, avocados, broccoli, leafy greens, nuts, seeds, soybeans, watermelon, cantaloupe, milk, legumes, fish, and dried fruit.

Increasing magnesium is also thought to lower blood pressure. Spinach, tofu, millet, pumpkin seeds, sunflower seeds, almonds, broccoli, wheat germ, blackstrap molasses, and lentils are all high in magnesium.

Last, sodium can dramatically increase blood pressure in people who are sensitive to its effects. Decrease salt consumption to less than 2,100 milligrams per day, or 1,500 milligrams per day for those over the age of fifty, African Americans, and those already diagnosed with hypertension. Use the Nutrition Facts on food labels to find foods options with less sodium.

More Heart Healthy Foods

For this week, try to eat some of these vitamin-B-rich foods at least once a day:

Folic Acid: Fortified/whole grains, legumes, sesame seeds, oranges, spinach, broccoli, wheat germ, Brussels sprouts, peas, avocado, dark green leafy vegetables, asparagus

Niacin (B_3): Chicken, fish, fortified/whole grains, red meat, peanuts

Riboflavin (B_2): Dairy products, clams, eggs, wheat germ, fortified/whole grains, mushrooms

Thiamin (B_1): Wheat germ, pork, fortified/whole grains, salmon, legumes, watermelon, pine nuts, okra, green peas

Vitamin B_6: Oatmeal, potatoes, avocado, wheat germ, prunes, fortified/whole grains, peanuts, bananas, garbanzo beans, lean meats/poultry, fish, sunflower seeds, and spinach

Vitamin B_{12}: Red meat, poultry, seafood, dairy products, eggs

Other food suggestions we've covered so far are also important to heart and vascular health:

- Avoid simple sugars and refined or processed grains to regulate insulin and control blood sugar; this improvement can then decrease "bad" cholesterol levels (LDL).
- Increase omega-3 fatty acids. Higher intakes of omega-3 fatty acids reduce blood clotting, lower triglycerides, and may also lower blood pressure. Omega-3 fatty acids can also improve cardiovascular health.
- Antioxidants, such as vitamin C, can help raise "good" HDL cholesterol levels.

- Substitute vegetables or soy foods for animal protein that is high in saturated fat.
- Eat more nuts. At least one ounce of nuts a day has been shown to reduce LDL cholesterol levels.
- Fiber, especially the soluble type, binds total cholesterol in the intestinal tract and promotes cholesterol excretion.
- Focus on low-glycemic-index foods. A moderate intake of low-glycemic-index foods has been shown to lower triglycerides and raise "good" cholesterol levels (HDL).
- Plant sterols and stanols are substances that occur naturally in many grains, vegetables, fruits, legumes, nuts, and seeds. Since they have moderate cholesterol-lowering properties, manufacturers have started adding them to foods, including margarine spreads (avoid any with trans fats), orange juice, cereals, and even granola bars. Studies have shown that two grams of stanol/sterol per day can significantly reduce LDL cholesterol.
- Eat garlic. The equivalent of one to two cloves of garlic a day has been shown to lower cholesterol levels and prevent blood clots.

Keep Thinking Green and Leafy

Spinach and other dark leafy greens show up on almost every list of foods that are good for you. They are high in B vitamins, antioxidants, omega-3 fats, potassium, magnesium, and fiber. Enjoy them raw or cooked, alone or as part of a recipe.

Broccoli and other cruciferous vegetables are not only a great source of vitamin C and beta carotene; they also contain phytochemicals known to be cancer preventive. Eat them raw or lightly steamed to retain the bulk of their antioxidant value.

Looking Forward to Success

In just thirty days, you may begin to think and feel differently. Physically, you might have more energy to exercise, your skin may feel suppler, and your hair might be shinier and healthier looking. You might even find that you are sleeping more soundly. If these eating suggestions were drastically different from the way you had been eating, you might be pleasantly surprised to see that you've lost a few pounds.

Internally, you may feel better. This is because with a high-nutrient diet, your immune function may improve as inflammation decreases. Over time, you may realize that you aren't getting as sick as often, or that you've seen improvements in your digestion.

You can expect to have more mental energy and improved cognitive function as well. It's much easier to stay focused and on task when you are eating properly. You might also feel less anxious if stubborn food cravings have ended. In fact, overall you can look forward to feeling content because you know that your brain and body are receiving the best raw materials in order to function optimally.

Chapter 7

THE 30-DAY
BRAIN HEALTH WORKOUTS

You may have heard that exercise is critical for keeping the heart and the rest of your body young. Exciting new evidence is now showing us how beneficial cardiovascular exercise can be for brain health as well. Study after study has shown that exercise may be one of the most important pillars of peak performance when it comes to taking care of your brain, because it has been directly linked to protecting and improving brain health as well as enhancing cognitive performance. This is true for all age ranges, from school-age children who want to perform better in the classroom to men and women looking to maintain their edge in the workplace to seniors who want to continue to lead vibrant and exciting lives, as well as those who might already be experiencing some form of cognitive impairment.

Exercise, more than diet, is neuroprotective. In a 2012 study with rats, exercise reversed high-fat-diet-induced cognitive decline. A second Japanese study demonstrated that mice that had been switched to a low-fat diet had fewer plaques and better memories than mice eating higher-fat fare. But what was even more interesting was that the mice in the group that were exercising had even healthier brains and better memory scores than the low-fat group—even when they had remained on a high-fat diet. In other words, exercise was more effective than diet control in terms of reducing high-fat-diet-induced Alzheimer's disease development. At this point, we can only guess that the results would be the same for humans. However, researchers believe, as we at Canyon Ranch do, that there's enough accumulating evidence about the potential cognitive risks of poor diet and the countervailing benefits from physical activity to recommend a cardiovascular program (as outlined in this chapter) for those looking to enhance their brain health.

You've already learned that brain function declines with underuse and age. Beginning in our late twenties, most of us will lose about 1 percent of the volume of the hippocampus every year. This area is a key portion of the brain related to memory and learning. We now know that exercise seems to slow or reverse the brain's shrinking, much as it maintains muscle mass. Research conducted at the University of Pittsburgh, the University of Illinois, Rice University, and Ohio State University has shown that regular cardiovascular exercise not only maintains the size of the brain but actually increases it, even in subjects in the fifty-five-to-eighty age range.

In a 2011 study released by the University of Arizona, researchers found that physically fit older men and women showed fewer age-related changes in their brains. And in this case, more is better: researchers found that the more physically fit individuals in the study had the fewest age-related brain changes. And for people who have already experienced losses in cognitive function, exercise has also been a key feature in reversing poor brain health. A 2010 study from the University of Washington School of Medicine documented that exercise improves cognitive performance in older adults with mild cognitive impairment (MCI) in as little as six months.

One of the reasons behind this phenomenon is that exercise is directly linked to neurogenesis. A 2010 study from the Salk Institute connected exercise to enhancing stem cell production in the brain, which is how new neurons are created. It was found that exercise "wakes up" dormant stem cells in the hippocampus to start making new neurons and improve memory. In animal studies, mice and rats that run for a few weeks generally show twice as many new neurons in their hippocampi as sedentary animals. Exercise also seems to make these new neurons nimble so that they can more easily connect into the neural network.

Best of all, research shows that it's never too late to start exercising for you to achieve these important benefits. In 2001, Danielle Laurin at the National Institutes of Health found that active women over the age of sixty-five were able to reduce their risk of dementia and Parkinson's disease with exercise. Compared with no exercise, physical activity was associated with lower risks of cognitive impairment, Alzheimer's disease, and dementia of any type. What's more, the study found there was a dose response: the more the women engaged in exercise, the better their results on cognitive testing.

At the same time, the most recent science shows that exercise doesn't have to be exhausting or painful to be effective, especially in terms of the brain. When a group of 120 older men and women were assigned to walking or stretching programs for a major 2011 study, the walkers were the ones who were able to produce increases in the size of their hippocampi after just one year; the stretchers lost volume to normal atrophy. The walkers also performed better on cognitive tests. The researchers concluded that the walkers had regained as much as two years of brain health simply by walking.

Exercise and physical activity can be categorized into four main types.

1. *Aerobic or cardiovascular exercise*: The movement of large muscles in a rhythmic way that results in elevation of heart rate. Examples include: walking, running, using the elliptical machine, biking, dance, and swimming.

2. *Muscle strength and muscle endurance training*: Working your muscles against some form of resistance, including: free weights, weighted machines, your own body weight, and resistance bands or tubing.

3. *Flexibility*: Commonly known as stretching, this includes most forms of yoga, Pilates, and traditional stretching exercises.

4. *Balance/coordination*: Activities that challenge one's balance/coordination.

For Better Brain Health, Focus on Aerobic Exercise

A 2012 study, part of the ongoing Memory and Aging Project at Rush University Medical Center in Chicago, was published in the journal *Neurology* and revealed findings that any type of movement has protective qualities for the brain. Muscle activities, such as resistance training, flexibility, stretching, and balance exercises, have all been shown to activate neurogenesis. However, aerobic exercise appears to be the most crucial for enhancing brain health. While a limited number of studies have found cognitive benefits among people who lifted weights, most studies to date, and all animal experiments, have involved running or other aerobic activities. The results of these studies are conclusive: consistent aerobic exercise allows you to preserve existing brain cells and grow new brain cells.

Aerobic training has also been successfully demonstrated to increase the production of three of the most important growth factors for neurogenesis. The first regulator for this process is a substance called *brain-derived neurotrophic factor*, or BDNF. This protein is produced in the skeletal muscles and brain cells and acts like a fertilizer for the brain: it aids in the growth of new neurons as well as improves the function of existing cells. BDNF strengthens the connections among neurons and protects brain cells from dying off; this means that when you produce more BDNF, you're able to hold on to your cognitive network longer. In fact, studies have shown that when BDNF is placed on neuronal cells outside the body, it keeps these neurons alive and multiplying. Cardiovascular workouts increase the production of BDNF, and these levels remain elevated for several hours afterward. Another very important finding is that engaging in a program of aerobic exercise for eight months or longer will teach the body to elevate its baseline BDNF level. This higher level then provides constant increased production of BDNF.

A second type of growth factor is *insulin-like growth factor 1* (IGF-1). This is a hormone produced in the liver that stimulates cell growth in tissues throughout the body, including the brain. Studies have shown that cardiovascular exercises can raise the number of new neurons created in the adult hippocampus because of an increased presence of IGF-1.

In addition, aerobic exercise increases blood flow to all parts of the body, including the brain, by improving vascular health. A third type of brain fertilizer is known as *vascular endothelial growth factor* (VEGF). VEGF is a naturally occurring protein that is critical for the growth of new blood vessels, and increases the oxygen supply throughout the brain and the body. Every new brain cell needs to be nourished with blood and oxygen. One exciting and surprising adaptation to consistent cardiovascular exercise is an increase in capillary density. VEGF has been shown to create new blood vessels in tissues that experience low oxygen levels or that are exposed to VEGF. As a result, skeletal muscles that are exercised and brain tissue that is exposed to VEGF can experience the growth of new blood vessels. Increasing capillary density in the brain also minimizes inflammation and slows down cell self-destruction, so this increase can help you retain memory and attention capabilities as you get older.

Last, we can't overlook the enormous benefits that aerobic exercise has for the rest of the body. It is an important component of a total health protocol that can be used preventively to help avoid a variety of diseases—including heart disease, obesity, and diabetes—that may influence brain health and certainly contribute to overall aging. For example, the risk of stroke is by far a more common brain health issue than the risk of Parkinson's disease. Because of this, improving your overall vascular health with regular aerobic exercise is directly connected to enhancing brain health. A 2011 study conducted at the Institute for Exercise and Environmental Medicine at Texas Health Presbyterian Institute Dallas suggested that for women age sixty and older, brisk walking for thirty to fifty minutes three or four times per week improved blood flow to the brain by as much as 15 percent. So even if you are thin, or if you're close to your ideal weight and are happy with the way you look on the outside, you still need to engage in cardiovascular exercise in order to stay healthy on the inside.

We've put together a thirty-day cardiovascular exercise program that is integral to maintaining and enhancing the brain as well as the body. But that's just the first step; while we think you'll see improvements during this time frame, we want to make sure exercise becomes part of your lifestyle now and going forward. Research shows that exercise-induced brain protection is lost once a regular exercise program is stopped. So no matter how long or how intensely you've been training, your body begins the detraining process just seventy-two hours after your last workout. In other words, cardiovascular exercise must become a part of your lifestyle in order for you to enjoy optimum brain health.

Strength Training and Depression

Strength training is an excellent way to help you maintain a positive self-image and avoid depression. Hundreds of studies have analyzed the effect of exercise on depression and found that strength training can raise self-esteem, enhance mood, reduce anxiety levels, increase the ability to handle stress, and improve sleep patterns. In one Brazilian study, sixty-five- to seventy-five-year-old men were able to improve mood and decrease anxiety after twenty-four weeks of strength training three times a week. Researchers discovered that during this time the men had increased levels of IGF-1, in much the same way as could occur with aerobic exercise.

GETTING STARTED

The best exercise prescription for the brain is a variable-intensity cardiovascular program, one that exposes your body to a variety of exercise intensities from day to day. The type of cardiovascular or aerobic activity you select is a personal choice. We suggest choosing several different activities to avoid boredom and injury. It is important to choose an exercise program that you enjoy and that does not produce pain in your body. As long as you can get the intensity up into the appropriate level, it does not matter what type of aerobic exercise you select.

If you are new to exercise, consider the following when selecting your types of cardiovascular activity:

- Do you prefer indoor or outdoor activity?
- Do you prefer group activity or solo activity?
- Do you prefer to exercise alone, with a small group of friends, or with a large group of strangers?
- Do you have pain or special orthopedic concerns that need to be taken into consideration?

KNOWING YOUR WORKOUT INTENSITY IS CRITICAL

To follow this program, you will need a tool to assess your exercise intensity or effort. This is critically important because exercise intensity is the main ingredient that affects brain health. During this program you will be working at three different intensities: low, moderate, and high.

By knowing your optimal training intensity, you will prevent yourself from working out too hard and subsequently hating your exercise program, while at the same time avoiding exercise intensities that are too low to create the desired improvement in brain health.

Each intensity level plays a role in optimizing brain health: the moderate-intensity exercise sessions have been shown to improve brain-derived neurotrophic factor (BDNF) and vascular endothelial growth factor (VEGF); the high-intensity sessions are associated with BDNF stimulation and the natural release of human growth hormone, which activates neurogenesis. Even low-intensity training can still have excellent effects on the biochemical adaptations that occur on the cellular level, and help to keep blood well oxygenated, thus decreasing the risk of arterial stress and damage.

While you may be completely motivated to jump right into a challenging exercise program, we recommend a more careful approach, especially regarding high-intensity exercise. Some studies suggest that when high-intensity exercise is performed before you have achieved a certain level of conditioning, it causes excessive oxidative stress in the body, which leads to free-radical production and inflammation. However, once you have achieved some baseline fitness, less oxidation occurs because the exercise effort is less stressful to the body and fewer free radicals are produced. This is why we do not recommend any high-intensity exercise (greater than 85 percent of maximum heart rate) until you have done at least six to eight weeks of base fitness building at the moderate and lower intensities.

We recommend using one of two tools or methods to measure and monitor exercise effort/intensity. One method is simple and low-tech, while the other involves the use of a heart rate monitor and is more complex. Both of the following methods work well; simply choose the method that works for you.

Heart Rate Monitoring

The most objective, scientific way of monitoring exercise intensity is through heart rate monitoring. This method requires knowing your target heart rate range and having a way to accurately measure heart rate during exercise. The best tool to precisely monitor heart rate during activity is a heart rate monitor. The type we recommend is called a chest-strap model and is by far the most common. These units feature two pieces: a transmitter chest strap and a wristwatch receiver. The chest strap picks up the electrical signal your body uses to fire the heart and relays this signal to the wristwatch for display. The chest strap should fit snugly around the upper chest and must be worn directly on the skin (under all clothing) just below the sternum. Be sure the strap maintains good contact with the skin or the heart rate will not be detected. Sweating, or the application of a small amount of water, normally improves the connection. Three heart rate manufacturers we recommend are Polar, Nike, and Garmin, and each makes several models that cover a range of sophistication and price points.

Rate of Perceived Exertion

An easier way to monitor your perceived exertion or rating of perceived exertion (RPE) during an aerobic activity is through estimation. In order to do this you need to periodically take inventory of how hard your leg muscles are working and what your breathing effort is like during activity. Then in your mind, combine these two feelings (leg effort and breathing effort) and rate your effort on the following scale, which is related to your maximum heart rate:

RPE Score	Feelings	% of Maximum Heart Rate
1–2	Sitting or standing still; no exertion at all	30–45%
3–4	Light movement; slight feeling of exertion	45%–65%; low
5–6	Moderate effort to slightly challenging	65%–75%; moderate
7–8	Challenging to very hard effort	75%–90%; high
9–10	Very hard to all-out maximal effort	90%–100%

Know Your Maximum Heart Rate Zone

In aerobic exercise, intensity can be measured in heartbeats per minute, or more particularly, what percentage of maximum heart rate you are working at. Your maximum heart rate is the highest possible heart rate you can achieve. It is an all-out 100 percent effort that is severely uncomfortable. Even the most fit, motivated athletes in the world can sustain this effort for only three or four minutes. During this or any other exercise program, you do not need to, nor should you ever, work out at your maximum heart rate.

In order to determine various percentages of maximum heart rate that are safe and effective to optimize brain health, you need to first figure out your maximum heart rate, using one of the following methods.

1. *A submaximal exercise test performed by an exercise physiologist:* During this test you will complete approximately fifteen

minutes of progressively more challenging exercise on your choice of equipment (treadmill, bike, elliptical, etc.) while wearing a chest-strap heart rate monitor. The workload of the exercise will increase every two minutes until you reach 85 percent of your maximum heart rate effort. Exercise physiologists are trained to use information such as breathing rate, speaking pattern between breaths, and perceived exertion to estimate an individual's 70 and 85 percent of maximum heart rate, and then they can mathematically calculate maximum heart rate.

2. *A VO_2 maximum test performed by an exercise physiologist:* This is the deluxe version of target heart rate determination. VO_2 stands for *volume of oxygen* consumed during exercise. During this test you wear a heart rate monitor in addition to a portable oxygen- and carbon-dioxide-measuring device called a *metabolic analyzer*. This device samples your expired breath and determines how much oxygen your body is consuming and how much carbon dioxide you are expiring during a graded exercise test in which the exercise intensity is increased steadily to 90 to 95 percent of maximal effort. This test reveals your optimal exercise heart rates as well as your aerobic fitness level (VO_2 maximum), your anaerobic threshold, and precisely how many calories you burn per minute at any given heart rate during exercise. This test is appropriate if you are at a low risk for heart disease.

3. *A cardiovascular stress test performed by a cardiologist:* The primary purpose of this test is to screen an individual for safe participation in cardiovascular exercise in terms of heart function and blood pressure tolerance. During this test you will have twelve electrodes placed around your heart. During the progressively harder exercise test, your physician will carefully watch your EKG tracing to see if your heart beats in a normal manner and if there is a lack of blood flow to

any parts of your heart. These electrodes also detect heart rate, so the physician can use your test results to estimate fairly accurately your maximum heart rate. Be sure to let your cardiologist know before the test that you want to learn what your maximum heart rate is, as the testers may need to slightly modify the protocol. This test is recommended for men over age forty-five and women over age fifty-five or those individuals at cardiovascular risk.

4. *Prediction equations:* Many published charts, heart rate monitors, and exercise machines (treadmills, bikes, or ellipticals) attempt to estimate maximum heart rate using age. In fact, any device into which you enter your age is most likely using your age to estimate your maximum heart rate. Unfortunately, this method has serious accuracy limitations. Any method that incorporates age into the estimation process is using an error-prone equation. However, for a very rough estimate of your maximum heart rate based on your age, you can use the following equation:

$$220 - \text{Age} = \text{Maximum Heart Rate}$$

Medications Can Affect Your Heart Rate

A family of drugs known as beta-blockers (which are commonly prescribed to control blood pressure and irregular heart beat) act by decreasing heart rate at rest as well as during exercise. Common beta-blockers are: Tenormin (atenolol), Lopressor and Toprol-XL (metoprolol), and Inderal (propranolol). If you are taking a beta-blocker, you should *never* use age-related calculations for target heart rate determination, as your heart rate will always be lower. Trying to achieve age-predicted heart rates can be impossible and potentially dangerous because these drugs can prevent your heart rate from increasing.

The 30-Day Brain Health Workouts

We have created three different monthlong workout programs to help you improve brain health. Whichever program you choose, we suggest sticking with it for the entire month, unless you are in physical pain or feel that it is unsustainable. The first is completely individualized, and is the best choice for beginners and first-time exercisers. The second program is more structured, and allows you to create an interval training program over the course of the month, so it is perfect for intermediate exercisers. The third option re-creates one of the most popular Canyon Ranch interval exercise programs right in your own home or at your local gym. This allows for interval training each day and is recommended for the intermediate or advanced athlete. This stepwise approach to exercise will limit injury and keep interest high—the two components necessary for an engaging and sustainable workout.

If you are planning on walking or running, you might want to invest in a device that measures movement, either a *pedometer* or an *accelerometer*. Some heart rate monitors come with these features. There are also some accelerometers that interface with software you can load on your computer or smartphone, including those by Fitbit, Nike, and BodyMedia. These devices can help with motivation and tracking your activity level.

Most important, before you begin any type of exercise program, please consult with your doctor and have a full physical. Once you have physician clearance to exercise, you can get started.

Choose Your Starting Fitness Level

Beginner Level

- New to exercise
- Have not exercised for more than three months
- Consider yourself to be out of shape

INTERMEDIATE LEVEL

- Currently doing three or fewer days per week of moderate to easy movement (golf, leisure walking, dog walking, etc.)
- Consider yourself to be active but not fit

ADVANCED LEVEL

- Currently exercise four or more days per week for forty minutes or more per session
- Currently doing some interval type of training
- Consider yourself to be fit

CHOOSE AN ACTIVITY

Pick at least one type of aerobic exercise that you will be able to engage in for the next thirty days. Afterward, you can continue with this type of exercise or change your program. However, you need to know that not all aerobic exercises are created equal: each utilizes a different amount of energy. The following table offers a way to standardize all types of exercise in relation to each other, in terms of how much energy they utilize. This table compares exercise *metabolic equivalents*, also known as METs. Whether you're sixty or thirty years old, if you cycle at ten miles an hour, it's the same MET score.

A MET is a measure of how much oxygen we use in a minute when we are just sitting or lying down. For example, a two-MET activity requires twice as much metabolic energy expenditure as resting. The maximum METs ($METs_{max}$) healthy people can achieve fall in the range of 7.1 to 22.9 METs, depending on a variety of physiological factors, including age, gender, genetics, overall health, and fitness level. The thirty-day goal is to get to a fitness level of at least seven METs if you are a man, and six if you are a woman.

METABOLIC EQUIVALENTS (METS) FOR AEROBIC ACTIVITIES

Beginners: Light-Intensity Activities	METs value
Football or baseball, playing catch	2.5
Stretching, mild hatha yoga	2.5
Walking, 2 mph, slow pace, firm surface	2.5

Intermediates: Moderate-Intensity Activities	METs value
Frisbee	3
Calisthenics, light or moderate effort	3.5
Trampoline	3.5
Bicycling, < 10 mph	4
Volleyball	4
Water aerobics, water calisthenics	4
Badminton, singles and doubles	4.5
Aerobic dancing, low impact	5
Walking, 4 mph, very brisk pace, firm surface	5
Ice-skating, 9 mph or less	5.5

Advanced: Vigorous-Intensity Activities	METs value
Bicycling, 10 to 11.9 mph, slow, light effort	6
Boxing, punching bag	6
Hiking, cross-country	6
Jog/walk combination (jogging component < 10 minutes)	6
Tennis, doubles	6
Aerobic dance class, moderate level, Zumba	6.5
Race walking	6.5
Jogging	7
Racquetball	7
Rowing machine	7
Ice-skating	7
Skiing	7
Soccer, casual	7

Advanced: Vigorous-Intensity Activities	METs value
Swimming laps, freestyle, moderate or light effort	7
Tennis, singles	7
Walking, backpacking	7
Basketball	8
Bicycling, 12 to 13.9 mph, moderate effort	8
Calisthenics, heavy vigorous effort	8
Football, touch, flag	8
Frisbee, ultimate	8
Rock or mountain climbing	8
Rope jumping, slow	8
Running, 5 mph (12 minutes/mile)	8
Snowshoeing	8
Boxing, sparring	9
Stairmaster, treadmill	9
Bicycling, 14 to 15.9 mph, racing, fast, vigorous effort	10
Judo, jujitsu, karate, kickboxing, tae kwon do	10
Rope jumping, moderate	10
Running, 6 mph (10 minutes/mile)	10
Swimming laps, freestyle, fast, vigorous effort	10
Rollerblading (in-line skating)	12
Squash	12
Running, 10 mph (6 minutes/mile)	16

RECORD YOUR PROGRESS

Use the following form to keep track of your exercise day by day, or plan ahead and follow along. Make several copies of this sheet, or create your own log in a notebook or journal, so that you can see your progress as you go. This log can be adapted for any of the three Canyon Ranch Brain Health Workouts.

Day/Date	Activity	Total Minutes	Maximum Heart Rate Level
Day 1			
Day 2			
Day 3			
Day 4			
Day 5			
Day 6			
Day 7			
Day 8			
Day 9			
Day 10			
Day 11			
Day 12			
Day 13			
Day 14			
Day 15			
Day 16			
Day 17			
Day 18			
Day 19			
Day 20			
Day 21			
Day 22			
Day 23			
Day 24			
Day 25			
Day 26			
Day 27			
Day 28			
Day 29			
Day 30			

The Individualized Canyon Ranch Brain Health Workout

If you are completely new to exercise, the first goal is to incorporate an aerobic workout into your daily schedule. Start by choosing an activity from the beginners' METs table, making sure that you can do that activity continuously for thirty minutes each day for five days. Do not break up your session: do all of your exercise at one time. Monitor your heart rate and make sure that you are working within 50 to 70 percent of your maximum heart rate.

On Day 6, immediately move to an activity from the intermediate category. At this point you have many more activities to choose from, and for the next fifteen days you can switch between exercises. Each day, make sure you are completing any one activity for twenty to forty minutes, with a day of rest once every five days, or on your rest days go back and choose an activity from the beginners' list. Again, do not break up your session: do all of your exercise at one time. Monitor your heart rate and make sure that you are working within 60 to 80 percent of your maximum heart rate. Record your progress and activity in the log.

On Day 21, move up to the advanced category of exercises only if you have reached an activity level that you are comfortable with. If you are enjoying the activities from the moderate category, you can continue to follow that routine, but work at an increased heart rate for a longer duration, extending your workout to sixty minutes. You can break up your session into two thirty-minute intervals during the course of the day. Continue to monitor your heart rate and make sure that you are working within 70 to 90 percent of your maximum heart rate.

Or choose an activity from the advanced category, and make sure you are completing the activity for twenty to forty minutes, with a day of rest once every five days, or on your rest days, go back and choose an activity from the beginners' list. Again, do not break up your session: do all of your exercise at one time. For activities in the advanced category, monitor your heart rate and make sure that you are working within 70 to 90 percent of your maximum heart rate.

On Day 31, congratulate yourself for a job well done. You have completed the individualized program and are now ready to move on to one of the other two brain health workouts. Or you can continue with your program at the advanced level. In thirty days, you may have created a new healthy habit that you can continue to support a lifetime of health and fitness.

The Structured Canyon Ranch Brain Health Workout

This is an introductory interval training program where you will be exercising at different intensities throughout the month, using the cardio activity of your choice from the intermediate or advanced METs table. The program is divided into three legs, each lasting ten days. By the time you get to the third leg of the program, you will be doing interval training every day.

- Days 1–10: During this stage you will focus on your base aerobic fitness. Work out at 60 percent of your maximum heart rate for forty to sixty minutes a day. You may break up the time into two sessions as long as the total is at least forty minutes. Do not take a rest day.

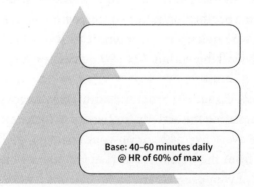

Base: 40–60 minutes daily
@ HR of 60% of max

- Days 11–20: During this stage you will introduce your muscles to a threshold workload that is higher in effort but still sustainable. The term *threshold* represents a 75 to 85 percent effort that can be maintained for a short amount of time. Using the same activities from the first ten days, every third day, work out for just twenty to thirty minutes at 75 to 85 percent of maximum heart rate. Do not take a rest day.

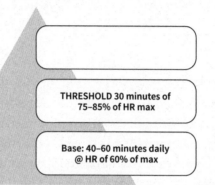

- Days 21–30: For the final stage of your thirty-day plan, you will begin to introduce the interval workout, which is characterized by efforts that exceed 85 percent of your maximum heart rate and cause fatigue, breathlessness, and a desire to slow down. These efforts above a level of 85 percent should last for only thirty to sixty seconds and should be followed by a two-to-three-minute recovery period, after which you can try the interval again. An example of this would be walking around a football field, then climbing the bleachers at a pace where you quickly become winded. Choose an activity from the METs table or use the same activities you have chosen in the past. Every day, work for just twenty to thirty minutes at 75 to 85 percent of maximum heart rate, including at least four to six interval efforts. Do not take a rest day.

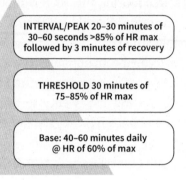

On Day 31, congratulate yourself for a job well done, and take a rest day—you've earned it. You have completed the structured program and can continue with this routine using any of the activities on the intermediate or advanced METs table. Or move on to the last of the brain health workouts. In thirty days, you may have created a new healthy habit that you can continue to support a lifetime of health and fitness.

The Canyon Ranch Stride Brain Health Workout

At Canyon Ranch we run a great treadmill class called "Stride," which is exceptionally popular. It's just like a spin class except it is performed on treadmills where incline and speed are regulated by the instructor. It's one of the best ways I know to guarantee a true interval training workout every day.

You can re-create a Stride class if you have access to a treadmill, either in your home or at a local gym. The following chart shows you the different intervals you'll be working in, based on time, incline, and speed. The goal is to follow along for the full workout for the next thirty days. If you cannot complete the entire workout, make sure that you complete the warm-up and cooldown sections.

On Day 31, congratulate yourself for a job well done, and take a rest day—you've earned it. You have completed the Stride program and can continue with this routine going forward. In thirty days, you may have created a new healthy habit that you can continue to support a lifetime of health and fitness. For a more vigorous workout, you can add 0.3 miles per hour to each speed throughout the program.

"STRIDE" WORKOUT

Time (in minutes)	Speed	Grade
WARM-UP		
0–1	2.5	0
1:00–2:00	2.8	0
3:00–4:00	3	0
4:00–5:00	3.3	0
MAIN SET		
5:00–6:00	3.3	4
6:00–7:00	3.3	0
7:00–8:00	3.3	4
8:00–9:00	3.3	0
9:00–10:00	3.3	4
10:00–11:00	3.3	0
11:00–12:00	3.3	5
12:00–13:00	3.3	0
13:00–15:00	3.3	3
15:00–17:00	3.3	0
17:00–19:00	3.3	4
19:00–21:00	3.3	0
21:00–23:00	3.3	5
23:00–25:00	3.3	0
25:00–28:00	3.3	3
28:00–30:00	3.3	0
30:00–33:00	3.3	4
COOLDOWN		
33:00–34:00	3	0
34:00–35:00	2.8	0
35:00–36:00	2.5	0

Get Your Groove On

Studies have shown that listening to music during exercise can improve results. Researchers have also found that some kinds of music are simply better to listen to than others, especially when it comes to creating a cardiovascular workout. Dr. Costas Karageorghis, an associate professor of sport psychology at Brunel University in England, found that the most important element in choosing the right music is tempo; the sweet spot is between 120 and 140 beats per minute, or BPM, which roughly corresponds to the average person's heart rate during a routine workout.

It turns out that this pace coincides with the range of most commercial dance music. The best workout songs have both a high BPM count and a rhythm to which you can coordinate your movements.

Sports and Activities That Enhance Brain Function

Certain sports are optimal for enhancing brain function beyond the scope of a strict cardio workout. These require a mix of speed, absolute attention, and *cognitive flexibility*, the ability to draw on diverse elements of knowledge to fit a particular need or problem-solving situation. Most often, these characteristics go hand in hand: if you choose an activity that might require some speed, you'll have to pay attention and be cognitively flexible.

The downside of running or walking on a treadmill is that even when you're doing it vigorously, your mind can wander to the things you're worried about. The following sports actually utilize different parts of the brain at the same time and create new neuronal connections. These factors are present at all skill levels, and increase and become more complex as you get better.

Tennis is a great example of a sport that combines all three elements—speed, absolute attention, and cognitive flexibility. First, it's a game where you have to react quickly, and eventually it will help you reduce your reaction time in a host of different environments off the court. There is a famous saying in neuroscience: "Neurons that fire together wire together." This refers to the fact that the more we repeat the same actions and thoughts—from practicing a tennis serve to memorizing how to conjugate verbs in a foreign language—the stronger the neural circuits in the brain for that activity become, decreasing your reaction time. This is sometimes referred to as *muscle memory,* but it actually takes place in the brain.

Tennis also requires you to pay total attention to the game. If you take your eyes off the ball, or even if you have a distracting thought, you'll lose that point. When you're playing tennis, your brain goes into a state of meditation: you have to maintain a single focus on "must get to ball, must get lower than that." While you're playing, you can't afford to think about an argument with your spouse or friend, or a project at work, or other worries in your life. Instead, you're stretching your mind, thinking only of that tennis ball.

Cognitive flexibility comes into the situation because in tennis, you have to know how to read your opponent, and if you are playing doubles, you'll need to figure out how to best work with your partner. In addition, Dr. Joan Finn at Southern Connecticut State University discovered that tennis players scored higher in optimism while scoring lower in anxiety and tension than other athletes and nonathletes.

Golf is another activity that requires complete focus, but not speed or cognitive flexibility. However, it's still a very good brain exercise. First, it requires visualization. By imagining your swing, putt, or overall form, you're exercising the right side of the brain, which is responsible for creativity. It also improves your coordination, whether it's hand-eye or balance as you complete your swing, and so it exercises your cerebellum—one of the areas of your brain responsible for coordination.

There is also some cognitive benefit from trying new activities in general. Taking any kind of dance class, from tango to Zumba, where you have to follow the instructions of a leader and learn new steps would fit the bill. Not only is dancing great exercise, increasing blood flow to the brain, it also improves your balance, coordination skills, and sense of timing/rhythm—all important facets of brain health. Dancing also enhances neurogenesis because you are creating new neural networks as you master new skills.

All of these suggestions have another huge advantage: There is a distinct social component to them. While it's great to do aerobic exercise every day, you also need to throw into the mix every once in a while an activity you must complete with somebody else. This will help keep mood up and depression down, and gets you out of your own head and your own house.

Chapter 8

---

30 DAYS OF MEDITATION, MINDFULNESS, AND SPIRITUAL CONTEMPLATION

Many of the mysteries of life are intricately connected to the mysteries of the brain. One of those areas is our inherent search for meaning—what we refer to as a spiritual quest. We don't fully understand why some people are more spiritually connected than others, and scientifically, we haven't been able to locate a specific area of the brain where spirituality takes place. However, we do know that people who engage in spirituality are happier overall and live longer lives. And we know that there are many areas of the brain that seem to be activated during spiritual contemplation, including part of the frontal lobe, the temporal lobe, and specifically the posterior temporal parietal area. Over time, these areas can become more developed as we engage in spiritual pursuits.

Meditation is one way to consciously exercise these parts of the brain. At Canyon Ranch we have found that through different spiritual practices, including meditation, many find that they connect with something larger than themselves. Your spiritual path is just one aspect of the process of discovering who you really are, as you learn to live in a place where your actions are in alignment with your true nature. If you already follow a spiritual path, meditation does not have to be separate from it. Instead, it is another way to connect with that path.

Your path does not have to be an organized religion, although it can be. At Canyon Ranch we don't focus on or support any particular religion. We do, however, encourage you to cultivate your own spiritual connection, and one way to do that is through meditation. What's more, you can also reap the benefits of meditation without attaching it to a spiritual journey. Everyone and anyone can learn to meditate and receive the full beneficial health effects, including the reduction of stress.

While an eating program and exercise regimen are parts of the work you need to do to maintain and enhance brain health, I like to think of meditation as more of a gift. It is one of the few daily activities where you can indulge in something that we all have very little of: time. Best of all, you are using this time to enhance all aspects of brain health as you relax and unwind after the hectic craziness of the day and connect deeply to what matters most to you.

The rewards that come with this gift are enormous. Meditation is one of the best-known tools for improving all four spheres of well-being—physical, mental, emotional, and spiritual. In the physical realm, scientific research shows that an ongoing meditation practice can lead to increased development of several key areas of the brain, especially those related to higher-order cognitive functions. It has also been proven to increase brain activity and improve attention and concentration. Studies on accomplished meditators—predominantly Buddhist monks—have shown that formalized meditation practice has allowed them to develop the ability to create a synchronized electrical rhythm throughout the brain that is unlike anything we normally see. In fact, their brain activity is typically different from ours in three distinct ways. First, brain waves in their cerebral cortex pulse in a distinct, unified fashion. They have also developed a profound ability to reduce their sense of pain by controlling the release of the brain's own pain reliever, endorphins. Last, their brains have the highest dopamine activation ever seen in terms of deriving pleasure from doing good deeds for others.

According to Jon Kabat-Zinn, PhD, of the University of Massachusetts Medical School, meditators can shift their brain activity to different areas of the cortex: for example, brain waves in the stress-prone right frontal cortex move to the calmer left frontal cortex. In other words, those who practice meditating can actually change their brain activity to make themselves calmer and happier. At the same time, researchers believe that when we meditate we *may* move from a chiefly left-brain dominance (verbal, cognitive, self-involved) to a more right-brain orientation (emotional, intuitive, inclusive). By doing so we focus our attention away from the nagging voice in our heads and toward a quieter, right-hemisphere state, which is where we can experience a feeling of connection and communion with things. This may be why many people who meditate report feeling "at one" or "connected" with the world. It's almost like taking a right-brain break from the ego-centric part of our lives.

Scientists also think meditation can assist in neurogenesis. In a 2009 study from UCLA's David Geffen School of Medicine, researchers used high-resolution MRIs to determine that long-term meditators had significantly larger gray-matter volumes in areas of the brain that are connected to emotional regulation and response control. This can mean that successful meditators are better able to control their stress levels, reducing anxiety and improving overall mood. As we know, these are key components for maintaining a sharp brain.

In the mental realm, meditation helps us to be present in all aspects of our lives, and this presence in turn allows us to become more aware and attentive. Zoran Josipovic, a research scientist and adjunct professor at New York University, believes as we at Canyon Ranch do, that meditation cultivates attentional skills. Dr. Josipovic's research is part of a larger program that is identifying a default network in the brain. His researchers are finding that the brain appears to be organized into two networks: the extrinsic network and the intrinsic, or default, network. The extrinsic portion of the brain becomes active when we are focused on an external task, whether it is raking leaves or studying for an exam. The default network controls our inner lives and is activated when we reflect on ourselves and our emotions. Dr. Josipovic has discovered that some Buddhist monks and other experienced meditators have the ability to keep both neural networks active during meditation. This ability may also define and explain the harmonious feeling of oneness with their environment that meditators report.

Many of us have a habit of living in our heads, where we have hundreds if not thousands of disparate thoughts going on all day. Unfortunately, we sometimes get entangled in all these thoughts; we occupy our minds very easily, and we determine that certain things are more real or more important than others. The benefit of meditation is that it brings peace into a mind that's spinning at a million miles an hour, allowing you to let go of as many distractions as possible and pay attention to a few thoughts at a time so you can have serenity. With practice, you'll be able to significantly quiet the mind and find a centered, sacred space you can return to whenever you want.

Emotionally, meditation quiets the mind and brings peace and tranquillity and a deep sense of contentment in life. It gives us the opportunity to relax and feel whole. When we're anxious, we may feel broken, or disconnected from those around us. In order to heal, we need to learn how to take care of ourselves when we know we're upset or stressed. Meditation is one way to focus on yourself so you can heal, as you learn to put the outside world aside and create a space in which you can experience your feelings without reacting to them or being consumed by them. You can acknowledge them with an attitude of self-acceptance and self-compassion. In the process, you can begin to make peace with yourself and feel more balanced and whole.

Unfortunately, most people are not honest with themselves. Instead, many are trying to run away from the past, relinquish control of the present, or close off their emotional lives. For example, some of the guests who come to the ranch tell us all the things they know they should be doing to improve their health. While we appreciate that they know what they could be doing, they're not letting themselves be honest with how they feel. Instead of saying, "I should be exercising more," an honest response would be, "I don't know why exercise is so hard to work into my daily routine. I'm really having a difficult time sticking to my program." Until you can actually accept your truth and be honest about what you're feeling, you'll find that it is very hard to move forward and create change. At Canyon Ranch, when we teach our guests how to meditate, we are also teaching them how to be true to themselves so they can tune in to the deepest part of their life and see how they are actually feeling. Finally, this sense of self-awareness and inner peace provides the perfect opportunity to explore spirituality.

Defining Meditation

There are many different kinds of meditation, each with its own slightly varied technique. Some require mental concentration. Others activate the imagination as it searches for peace or satisfaction. Meditation has also been described as taking a moment to sit quietly or to ponder. Regardless of the technique, the outcome is often the same: to slow down the incessant activity of the mind. Meditation brings a state of profound, deep peace that occurs when the mind is calm and silent yet completely alert.

Meditation is not an act of doing—it is a state of awareness or simply being. You can be meditating in your office as effectively as if you were sitting in the lotus posture on top of a mountain. The point is not to be attached to what's happening on the outside, but to focus on the inside. So setting is not that important.

During the next month, you'll be introduced to four different types of meditation. In the first week, you'll learn how to master the basic building blocks of a meditation practice—the tools you'll need to draw on. As the weeks progress, your practice will get deeper, and you'll be guided to think about bigger life issues you may need to resolve.

Don't put too much pressure on yourself to master meditation in this first month. If anything, meditation is an exercise in patience. Many people come to the ranch and expect to master meditation in a session or two, and they become frustrated when they don't. The typical response we hear is, "I tried meditation but it didn't work for me. My mind just kept going and going."

The truth is, this is exactly what is supposed to happen when you first begin to meditate, because that is the nature of the mind. That's why we call it a "meditation practice," because it takes time to learn how to quiet the mind. And just because your mind may wander, it doesn't mean that meditation isn't working. Instead of getting frustrated, realize that every day you practice, you are laying the foundation for making meditation a part of your lifestyle. Think of this month as the very first steps toward change.

Practice Makes Perfect

When you first learn how to meditate, you may actually feel more agitated instead of relaxed because you may be getting in touch with what you're really feeling for the very first time, and it might bring up negative or difficult emotions. This is actually very healthy. And as you practice and become more in tune with your authentic self, you'll be able to release some of your pent-up energy and relax. Over time, you'll learn how to quickly tap into your place of peace.

Some of this may seem like hard work, and you will be able to do it on your own. However, if you want to explore healing from past wounds or traumas, we recommend that you work with a skilled practitioner who can guide you.

THE PRACTICE OF MEDITATION

You can meditate wherever you are most comfortable. Sit in a chair or on a couch. You can sit cross-legged or with your feet flat on the floor. Make sure to hold your head and neck upright. If you find that you are too restless to sit in meditation, get up and take a walk, do a chore, or run an errand. Then come back and try again. Usually you'll feel calmer and more able to relax.

We suggest that you wear comfortable, nonbinding clothing and find a quiet space where you can turn off as many distractions as possible. Some people like to create a special place in their home to meditate. We don't suggest meditating on a bed—you might fall asleep—or in a room filled with other people (unless you are engaging in group meditation).

Some people like to meditate in silence. Others enjoy listening to soft music or chanting. Sleep music that features the sounds of waves or rainfall or other natural rhythms can also be effective. You might also like to record yourself reading aloud the instructions for the individual meditations below so you can play them back during your practice.

It helps if the lights are dimmed. Some people like to light candles during their meditation. If you are so inclined, we recommend using them safely: always place candles on a flat, fire-resistant surface, such as a ceramic dish.

Creating Your Meditation Space

Do you have a room or a space inside or outside your home where you can meditate? It doesn't have to be fancy, as long as you can make it beautiful and make it your own. If you are creating a mediation space, surround yourself with objects that help you feel peaceful and comfortable. You can evoke that feeling with a beautiful painting or photograph, some flowers, a seashell, or a religious symbol. The space could be as simple as a room with a great view or a spot in your living room or den where you can focus on a favorite painting or photograph. It could also be as small as an altar that houses a collection of your favorite things or as simple as a beloved meditation cushion.

Once you're in your space, unplug. No TV, no cell phone, no computer. The point is to carve out some time for quality silence.

WEEK ONE: BASIC MEDITATION

For the first week, you will practice meditation for as little as ten minutes or as long as thirty minutes. Give yourself at least ten minutes to begin your practice. As you get deeper into the month, you may use up to forty-five minutes or an hour. You can revisit these basic exercises at least once a day, or whenever you feel the need to quiet your mind.

You may find it easier to meditate at a specific time, or times, each day. Many people find that early in the morning, before they get pulled into the activities of the day, is a good time. Meditating in the morning also helps to set a tone for the day. Of course, if you prefer to meditate later in the day or if your schedule requires it, then go with what works best for you.

You'll begin each meditation by closing your eyes and focusing attention on your breathing—following the inhalation and the exhalation. Let your breathing be slow, full, and rhythmic. This focus does not concern thinking about breathing so much as it concerns experiencing the sensation of breathing.

As you meditate, notice when your attention is drawn to a thought, sound, sensation, or emotion. Simply allow the experience to be there without resisting it, then gently bring your attention back to the breath. If you find yourself judging any aspect of what you are experiencing— for instance, if you find yourself lost in thought and judge this as "wrong" or "bad"—just notice the judgment as "thought" and bring your attention back to the breath.

What's most important is that you try to stay in the present. If what you are experiencing is pleasant and you notice any tendency to want to hold on to that experience, just let it go by returning to the breath. If what you are experiencing is unpleasant and you notice any tendency to push it away, just notice what you are experiencing and return to the breath. Remember, we are not trying to get anywhere when we meditate. We are practicing the art of being here.

Meditation Tool #1:
Breathing

When we're under stress, we move less oxygen to the brain because we inhale and frequently forget to exhale—unconsciously, we tend to hold our breath or breathe much more shallowly. One key to reducing stress is then to bring consciousness to your breathing. And so, if you really want to access your full brainpower, you need to make sure you're breathing more deeply and more consciously, especially before you need to remember something (to decrease anxiety).

Breathing for meditation means that you are bringing awareness to your breathing. We're breathing all the time without thinking about it.

If you want to experience the real benefits of meditation, then it helps to develop a conscious breathing practice. This can include counting, combining meditation with breathing, following a yoga practice, or just taking some time to carefully breathe on your own. You can also experiment with breathing through the nose as well as through your mouth.

It's a misconception that the practice of focusing on your breath allows you to empty your mind. Instead, you are focusing your attention on just your breath, and by doing so, you're developing an ability to pay exquisite attention to one thing. Paying attention to your breathing is a wonderful way to cultivate the ability to stay focused. For example, when you're surfing the Internet, you're distracted and at the same time stimulated by all these different pop-ups and colorful ads that are meant to grab your attention. It's easy to pay attention to every new thing that bursts in front of you, but it's hard to focus on just your breathing.

Breathing for meditation involves the ability to slow down or control your breathing. You want your breathing to be rhythmic and full. Breathing is a perfect focal point during meditation because it's already happening: you can't stop it. It will happen no matter what else you do without adding another complicated aspect to meditation, like a mantra. Because your breathing is happening right now, focusing on it helps you to keep your attention rooted in the present.

At Canyon Ranch we teach a variety of breathing techniques and simple meditations. Try all of them this week and see which you are most comfortable with.

4-4-8 Count Breathing

1. Sit in a comfortable position. You can also lie down, but you may be more likely to fall asleep. Close your eyes so that you don't get distracted by visual things.

2. Breathe in through the nose with your mouth closed for four counts.

3. Hold your breath for four counts.

4. Exhale through the nose or mouth for eight counts.

5. Repeat this practice for four minutes, then take a break; otherwise you may feel dizzy from holding your breath.

Deep Belly Breathing

1. Lie down or sit in a comfortable position with your eyes closed. Gently rest your hands on your stomach, to bring more awareness to this area.

2. Start inhaling through the nose, allowing the belly to extend fully. You will feel your hands rise.

3. Exhale through the mouth or nose, allowing the belly to contract.

4. Continue to do this breathing as long as you want.

Meditation Tool #2:
Progressive Relaxation

Progressive relaxation is a technique developed to reduce anxiety. We find it to be an effective mechanism if you are having difficulty falling asleep or as a beginning practice in meditation. During the exercise, you will be alternately tensing and relaxing the muscles of your body. The muscles are tensed for ten seconds and then relaxed for twenty seconds before moving to the next muscle group. The whole session can take up to thirty minutes.

1. Start by sitting or lying down in a comfortable position with your eyes closed.

2. Bring an awareness to your breathing. Begin by inhaling through the nose and exhaling through the mouth or nose.

3. Tighten your toes and then relax them.

4. Move up to your ankles and tighten them and relax.

5. Move up to your calves and tighten them and relax.

6. Continue up your body, tightening and relaxing each muscle group until you reach the top of your head. Then cycle back from the top of your head to your toes. This will help quiet the mind and ground you with a focus on your feet.

WEEK TWO: WALKING THE LABYRINTH

The second week moves to a more advanced type of meditation, known as *guided imagery*. It is meant to calm down the busy mind. You may want to record yourself very slowly reading aloud the following passage, so that later you can close your eyes and follow along. Or have someone you love read this for you to enhance your experience. Just as with the meditations for the previous week, you will want to set some time aside

The Soul Journey

One of our signature services is called Soul Journey. This individualized experience features a skilled practitioner who privately guides a meditation that helps you gain insight and intuition in order to facilitate healing. On the journey, you may be transported to a higher state of consciousness, awareness, and understanding. We find that this particular meditation is especially useful for those who are searching to find the beauty of their own lives.

for this exercise, wear comfortable nonbinding clothing, and find a space in your home where you will not be interrupted. You can revisit this guided meditation each day for one week, or whenever you feel the need to find your truth.

This meditation is based on a labyrinth we created at the Canyon Ranch in Lenox, Massachusetts. A labyrinth is an ancient meditation path. It has a spiral pattern, and its circles are feminine, nurturing, and filled with inner peace. They create a sense of being rather than doing. Typically, guests approach the labyrinth, and before they enter, they take a moment to relax and reflect. As they walk slowly to the center, they release concerns and quiet the mind. Once they reach the center, they stop to listen and pray, receiving what the moment offers. Then they walk their inspirations and intentions back out and resume their day, reflecting on what they experienced.

If you have access to a physical labyrinth, take this meditation with you. If not, you can create a labyrinth in your mind. Record the following, or have someone read it to you slowly as you enter your place of peace. If you are sitting or lying down, you can begin this time of meditation by allowing your eyes to close. Feel the support of the surface beneath your body and let yourself relax into it.

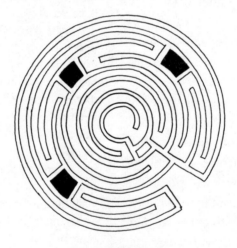

A LABYRINTH

Imagine yourself walking along a path that's lined by trees on either side. You come to a bridge that crosses over a gentle stream. Just ahead you see a labyrinth . . . an intricate circle of stones. The labyrinth is an ancient form that has been re-created by people of various cultures all around the world. It is a sacred place of healing, of wholeness. It is a place where you can walk your path, your journey, to connect deeply with yourself and all that is important to you—what truly matters. This is a space where you can connect with your hopes and your dreams for yourself and for those you love. This is your path, your journey.

As you enter the labyrinth, the experience is like going through a gate, a threshold, into a magical space, filled with a powerful vibrant energy. The air feels different here; it's charged, like the air near the ocean or on a mountain peak. The air is alive with energy and possibility. Breathe it in, feeling that energy filling you and connecting you with your deepest source of inspiration.

Begin following the circular path. As you make the first turn and walk the first ring, you can feel your connection to the earth. With each step, feel the earth beneath your feet; feel the strength and energy in your body. Reflect for a moment on the ways you nourish your body: eating healthy food, drinking pure fresh water, fortifying yourself with essential vitamins and minerals. You are feeling good and strong. Choose to nourish yourself with substances that support your health and well-being. Value your body and your brain, the source of your intelligence and your creativity, and make good choices that protect and fortify your brain. Value yourself and your health, and be fully present to the ones you love. Full, loving attention, all that you can be. Clear and vibrant, fully present with love and care. Find the sparkle in your eye; be able to fully enjoy the many blessings in your life.

And now make your turn into the next ring of the labyrinth . . . enjoying the feeling of moving forward, making progress, feeling the energy and vitality in your body, and knowing that this movement, taking time each day to move, to exercise, gives you strength and energy, brightens your spirit, and fortifies your health. You can see and feel yourself exercising, the rhythm of your movements, the energy coursing through your body, and know that you are stronger for this. Your mind is clearer, sharper, better able to focus your attention, to learn and to remember.

Make the next turn and, moving into another ring of the labyrinth, feel your breathing. Focus on the slow, deep, rhythm of it and enjoy the freedom to breathe deeply, to breathe fully, and to feel the relaxed energy that fills you with every breath you take. Your breath connects you with yourself, with a deep source of peace and strength that lives within you. Wherever you are, wherever you go, your breath can be a source of calmness, a constant companion that you can turn to again and again for strength, for confidence, and for comfort. The full, deep inhale, the long, slow exhale. Calm, peaceful, relaxed energy. Breathing in vitality, life energy that flows into every cell of your brain and body.

Make your way into the center of the labyrinth. This is the still point that exists right here in the present, in this moment, the only moment there is. Connect with the core of yourself, a deep source of knowing, a profound source of peacefulness, eternal and unchanging. The essence that remains constant through all the changes in your life. You have so many thoughts that arise in your mind, choices to consider, physical sensations, emotions that come and go. Every day, so many different thoughts, sensations, and feelings. And yet through it all, there is a strong, peaceful center of awareness within your that is eternal and unchanging.

And from this place of awareness, you can experience the fullness of the present moment. The richness of your emotions, the joy, the sadness, the comfort of a gentle touch, the beauty that surrounds you.

Connect with that strong, peaceful center of awareness. Clearing a space, a time that is just for you. A time outside of time. And connecting with that deep, strong, peaceful center of awareness inside you. From that center you can witness the flow of thoughts that arise in your mind. And you can observe them without becoming caught up in them; you can see them for what they are—just thoughts and not reality. Your mind is continually generating thoughts . . . thoughts about the past, concerns about the future—that is the nature of the mind. And yet there is that changeless place from which you can observe your thoughts and know that you are more than your thoughts, you are more than your emotions, and you are more than the physical sensations you experience in your body.

From this place of awareness, you can observe your thoughts— the judgments you make about yourself and others, the judgments you make about life. The things you worry about, the things that make you angry, and the things you regret and wish had never happened. From your mindful center of awareness, you can see the judgments of your mind for what they are. They are just thoughts, and not reality. And from this place of mindful awareness you can observe your judgments and choose to let them go. And so you are becoming more and more free, more and more able to determine how you respond to the events of your life . . . and all the while your compassion for yourself and others is deepening, becoming a growing acceptance of who you are and an appreciation that others are doing the best they can.

And now leave the center, making the turn into the next ring of the labyrinth and connecting deeply with what is most important to you. What you love and what you value. Thinking about what you cherish most: your health, your family, your friends, your good work. Thinking about what brings you joy and the energy you put into it. Taking a moment to savor what gives your life meaning and what you deeply appreciate.

Make one more turn, entering the last ring of the labyrinth, moving forward and feeling the strength to handle whatever life brings you. With each step, feel a new connection to your core, to who you are. Feel the strength of your resilience, your ability to face challenges, bounce back from adversity. And know that you are stronger for facing the challenge, for dealing with what life has given you; and know that nothing in your life is wasted, that every experience enables you to grow in wisdom and maturity, in your capacity to love and to dedicate yourself to what you care deeply about.

You have arrived at the gate once again and are standing at the threshold. Preparing to leave the labyrinth and carry with you what you have experienced here, holding in your heart what you have felt and learned about yourself. Walk through the gate and over the bridge that crosses the stream, knowing that you will continue on the path of your life and that you are stronger for this and that you can return to this place again and again and again.

Take a few deep breaths, breathing in energy and feeling that energy flowing into every part of your body. Flowing into your chest and abdomen, down your arms and into your fingers, down your legs and into your feet and toes, and up through your neck and into your head and face. And begin gently and gradually to open your eyes, coming into a place where you are feeling refreshed, feeling alert, and bringing the fullness of what you have experienced with you as you enter into this moment and as you enter into the rest of this day.

Connecting with Nature

One of the amazing things about Canyon Ranch is our connection and commitment to nature. Each of our properties is set in an extraordinary location, from the breathtaking Sonoran Desert to the placid beauty of the Berkshire Hills. As hard as it may seem to believe, I find that our guests become more balanced within minutes of being in nature. That's because when we return to nature, we feel an overall sense of connectedness.

WEEK THREE: THE SPIRIT WALK

Another benefit of meditation and spiritual practice is the ability to truly heal from personal wounds that may be holding us back from achieving what we want from our lives. Effective meditation can bring the practitioner a deeper spiritual connection, as you realize that the positive feelings associated with it are there for you always, and can be called on whenever you need them. Once you tap into that sense of connection, you will be able to heal.

This insight is especially valuable for anyone faced with addiction. As we discussed in chapter 3, addictive behaviors are a response to an imbalanced release of the neurotransmitter dopamine. This brain chemical is responsible for many things, including the rush that accompanies the feeling of reward or satisfaction. Any type of addictive behavior, whether it's to cigarettes, alcohol, sex, gambling, shopping, or a prescription or illegal drug, begins with the release of that first incredible dopamine rush. For some, this experience is so powerful it causes them to continually search for more of whatever turns them on. Yet each time you have another experience, you are rewarded with less dopamine. This is when the cycle of addiction begins: your brain is sending a signal, encouraging you to seek out more of that particular experience so that it can push out enough dopamine to give you that feeling of reward. So every time you are looking for new shoes, you can't buy just one pair, you buy two.

Luckily, it's possible to break an addictive cycle, especially when you begin to take care of your brain health. One of the most powerful ways is by deepening your connection with your spiritual side. Every 12-step program, including Alcoholics Anonymous, is at its core a spiritual journey from acceptance to recovery.

At the Canyon Ranch in Tucson, Arizona, we have created our own spiritual journey. It's called the Spirit Walk, and it consists of a moving meditation, literally. Instead of requiring you to sit in a room, this mental exercise takes place on an actual path and is accompanied by a set of questions to think about as you walk along a route to six separate locations on the property. Each of these locations is meant to inspire profound self-reflection and deep spiritual contemplation. One of the reasons why the Spirit Walk works so powerfully is that it is in nature. It is just one of many opportunities for our guests to get in touch with their natural state, to be outdoors in silence.

You can create your own Spirit Walk by marking out a trail where you can stop at least twice. At these stops, begin to reflect on the questions and thoughts below as if each were its own meditation. Take on one of the six main topics each day. By the end of six days, you will have completed one cycle of the Spirit Walk. On the last day, take a long walk and reflect on all the questions at once. You can revisit this Spirit Walk—in pieces or as a whole—whenever you feel the need to regroup. May your best intentions become realities as you begin your journey of self-discovery.

1. Reflection

What is my mission and purpose in life?

Many times, people fill their lives with things they are good at but don't really love doing. They might think, "I need to work in this shop for another ten years even though I hate it, because I want to make enough money to retire." A more fulfilling life will happen when you discover what really matters to you, and then figure out how to align with it and move toward your goals.

What do I want to release to create space for the new?

Are you in a transition? This can be anything from switching a job to getting divorced to getting married to wanting to lose weight (or improve your brain health) to having your kids move away from home to turning fifty (or sixty or seventy or eighty). Give yourself time to think about what you need to let go of to create the space for allowing the transition to take place.

2. Spirit

Where do I find spirit in my life?

Sometimes people think spirituality means meditation or prayer, but it can really be anything that allows you a sense of peace and connection. It can also be gardening. It could be dancing in your living room. Many people say that they find their spiritual connection in nature. Whatever helps you to feel connected can be considered spiritual practice.

Can my spirit motivate me to make a change to a healthier, more balanced lifestyle?

In order to let your spirit make these changes, you have to slow down so you can hear the true guidance of your intuition. Your intuition is your spirit. If you are really listening to what's there, then you will be able to achieve positive, enhancing changes in your life.

3. Peace

What would it take for me to be at peace in my life?

In order for peace to come, you have to be patient. Recognize what you can be grateful for right now. Accept the things you can't change. And learn to be patient with both yourself and others.

Are there people I'm ready to forgive? Can I forgive myself?

Follow this timeless Hawaiian teaching called *Ho'oponopono*. It is based on four tenets centered on a single concept: we each take 100 percent responsibility for our actions, for the actions of others toward us, and for everyone else as well. Review these four declarative statements until you find peace with whatever issue you may be struggling with, whether it involves another person or something about yourself that deserves forgiveness.

1. I'm sorry: Bring to the mind's eye those with whom you have an issue and tell them that you are sorry.

2. Please forgive me: Imagine an infinite source of love and healing flowing from yourself to these others, and ask for their forgiveness as you let your love and healing overflow out of your heart to them.

3. Thank you: When we are in a state of gratitude, we receive blessings.

4. I love you: Let go of the others, and see them floating away. If you have forgiven them, you will think of them without feeling any negative emotions. Let them know that you are sorry for your negative thoughts.

4. Serenity

In what areas of my life do I experience contentment and ease?

The only way you can achieve serenity is by being honest with yourself. Take a candid self-assessment to see where you are in harmony and where you are feeling stress. Bring awareness to that place where you're stressed, instead of avoiding it. Reprogram your brain to accept the challenges you face so you can appreciate the ease. Then acknowledge the places where you really do have contentment, instead of always focusing on the negative.

What do I wish for myself and for my loved ones?
Sometimes, people forget what really matters. Love, giving and receiving, your service to others, and your relationships are more important than all the things you can't take with you.

5. Intention

What decision have I been avoiding that I now want to make?
Sometimes we hold ourselves back from accepting change and being able to flow with it. Many people won't make a decision because they're afraid they'll make a mistake. Either they're terrified of the unknown or they're scared that their entire life is going to change. But the truth is that life is change. How else can we grow? We embrace the feeling of aliveness when we accept and allow for change.

What one promise that I'm willing to keep can I make to my true self?
Sometimes we take on more than is reasonable for us. Think about taking things one step at a time and making one commitment at a time. Wait until one step is complete before you allow yourself to take another. This is the true path to success and the way to think about making lasting change.

6. Discovery

How are recovery and discovery related for me?
Many of us live by the decisions other people are making for us. When that happens, we can get led off course from our own place of contentedness and peace. Recovery and discovery allow us to decide for ourselves, "Who am I?"

How have I let fear hold me back from living fully?
Making a mistake is not the worst thing in the world. And if you make a mistake, you can forgive yourself without the expectation of perfection. Next time, choose to trust your intuition instead of letting fear hold you back.

WEEK FOUR: MINDFULNESS MEDITATION

Another type of meditation is the practice of *mindfulness*, paying full attention to your present-moment experience with an attitude of curiosity and openheartedness. In essence, mindfulness practice is about learning how to pay attention. As simple a concept as it seems, the brain needs to practice the skill of concentration, and it takes work and discipline to develop strategies to stay focused. We usually regard this as part of growing up: we know that young children are very distractible, and as they get older, they have a better ability to focus on one task at a time. But our culture makes it harder for both kids and adults to develop attentional skills.

Our multitasking habits work because the brain needs—and is rewarded by—new stimulation. The brain is always looking for the next new thing, searching for any new piece of information. The excitement you feel when you see something new is actually the same release of the neurotransmitter dopamine that's implicated in addiction—it's a burst of energy that starts in the brain and, depending on how much it affects you, can travel throughout your body. That's why many of us find highly edited movies so compelling and why websites are designed with movement and blinking images: they grab your attention and force out a little squirt of dopamine so you'll feel the reward and you'll want to engage even more with the movie or the website. And people don't call BlackBerries "CrackBerries" for nothing. They're addictive, and again, the addiction is related to the dopamine reward. Every time you hear that little ding or see your phone flashing to tell you there's an e-mail, the brain responds by making you think, "What am I missing?"

Those are some of the reasons why we are unintentionally training our brains to receive all this data, and consequently, our attention span is becoming equally choppy. To counteract this, we need to practice the skill of being mindful, which lets you put everything else aside so you can focus on what you're choosing to be doing in the moment. Instead of looking for more stimulation, you're teaching the brain to focus.

Ram Dass talked about mindfulness in the 1970s in his famous book *Be Here Now, Remember,* yet its origins can be traced to 2,500 years earlier, to the teachings of the Buddha. Today, research shows that mindfulness is more than a theory; it is a very powerful approach to living that enhances brain function. When people cultivate mindfulness, their thinking becomes sharper. They're less distracted; they're less preoccupied with extraneous thoughts. What's more, a mindfulness practice can change the structure of the brain, encouraging neurogenesis. It also trains the brain so you can pay attention better, improve memory, decrease stress, and increase overall happiness.

In a 2011 study from Massachusetts General Hospital, researchers found that in just eight weeks, subjects who practiced a mindfulness meditation program were able to make measureable changes in brain regions associated with memory, empathy, and stress. The observed brain changes occurred during periods of meditation, but the benefits lasted throughout the day. Other studies have confirmed these findings. A study from the University of Pennsylvania taught a mindfulness practice to marines just before they were deployed to Iraq. Researchers found that these men and women performed better in the stressful situations of combat: they had a lower incidence of post-traumatic stress, and they performed better on cognitive tests than those who had not been given the mindfulness training.

Cognitive function improves with this type of meditation as well. A study completed at Wake Forest University on the cognitive effects of mindfulness meditation training found that after just four sessions of meditation training, participants with no prior meditation experience showed significant improvement in their visual-spatial processing, working memory, and executive functioning. These findings have been confirmed in other studies, including studies of participants who were beginning to exhibit the early signs of dementia.

The signature trait of mindfulness training is to increase your capacity to observe everything within and around you. By doing so, the practice of mindfulness keeps you from being *mindlessly* swept away by emotions, worries, or preoccupations. It also helps to keep you from snapping to conclusions or making judgments. For most people, not worrying about the past or not thinking about the future allows them to experience pleasure and satisfaction, the necessary components of happiness.

Another reason many of us become unhappy is that we have trouble accepting what is actually going on in our lives. With a mindfulness practice, you can become very good at noticing the judgments you automatically or habitually make, and by recognizing them, you can begin to free yourself from them. If you tend to be hard on yourself, mindfulness is a wonderful way of learning to be kinder to yourself. If you tend to be overly critical of other people, mindfulness can help you to notice those judgments and develop a better attitude of kindheartedness.

These improvements in attention and mood naturally foster better learning and memory. When we are anxious, we can get tripped up in conversation or forget what we were going to talk about or even lose the name of the person we are talking to. But if you practice mindfulness, you might shore up your own feelings of competence, which will lessen your anxiety. You'll have the confidence that you can follow a linear thought from the beginning of a conversation to the end, or remember names better because you are paying closer attention. As we like to say, "Better attention leads to better retention."

Most memory problems are really, at their source, attention problems. Problems arise when the information for creating new memory never gets encoded or stored in the first place. Mindfulness teaches you how to be in the moment, so you are better able to process information and solve problems. At the same time, when you learn to pay closer attention, your memory can naturally improve and your cognitive abilities may flourish.

A Formal Mindfulness Practice

There exist both a formal and an informal mindfulness practice. The formal practice consists of structured experiences like the meditations discussed in Week One. During the meditation, you will be asked to pay attention to many things: what's coming in through your five senses (what you're seeing, hearing, tasting, touching, and smelling); your kinesthetic experience (how your body is feeling: heaviness, lightness, tension); your thoughts; and your emotions.

A formal mindfulness meditation involves sitting in a comfortable, centered position and focusing your attention on just one thing. This focal point could be your breath, a mantra, or an image. The goal is to let the mind rest on just one stimulus. When the mind wanders away from the focal point and other things come into your awareness, notice them with an attitude of openhearted acceptance, and then come back to your focus again. Try to acknowledge the thought, but then let it go so you can return to your focal point.

For example, if you are sitting comfortably, with your eyes closed, and focusing on your breathing, thoughts might drift into your consciousness, such as, "I wonder who's going to show up at the meeting at three o'clock. Did I put that check in the mail? What am I going to serve my in-laws for dinner?"

Instead of pursuing these lines of thought, simply acknowledge them as, "I just had a thought." And then, gently let them go and come back to your breathing. The idea is not to engage in "thinking as usual." Instead, the goal is to quiet your mind and become more aware of the process of awareness itself. You can observe thoughts when they arise, without pursuing them or worrying about their content. You gently put them aside and return to your focal point.

Practice this formal mindfulness meditation for fifteen or twenty minutes each day. If you're short on time, you could do it in five minutes. Afterward, you don't need to write down the thoughts that came into your head, because they're really not important (unless you've just solved world peace: write that one down). By doing so, you're developing the skill of paying attention on purpose.

When you are faced with an issue of real importance, you'll find that you are better prepared to focus on it clearly. For example, when you're in a meeting, or you're talking to your kids or your spouse, and there are other distractions happening, you'll be able to consciously say to yourself, "I'm going to let that go so I can give this conversation my full attention . . . and then I'll deal with this other stuff later."

The Informal Mindfulness Practice

In addition to the formal practice, there's a host of informal practices you can do in any moment of your day:

- You're waiting in line at the grocery checkout, and you begin feeling impatient. You start thinking, "I'm so hungry and I have to make dinner, and now I have to wait in line." Instead, you can use mindfulness to look at the situation differently. You can breathe deeply and accept that you can't control how fast the line moves; what you can control is how you react. By openheartedly accepting the reality of the situation, even though you would not prefer it, you will feel less stressed waiting in line, and you'll feel calmer when you get home.

- You're having an argument with somebody you love, and you're judging this person. You can choose to be mindful at that moment and free yourself to look at the situation in a different way. You can mindfully observe the thoughts and feelings you are having in reaction to what your loved one is saying, and then choose to be less judgmental by trying to understand his or her feelings and position—and your own reactions to them, rather than being emotionally hijacked by your initial knee-jerk reaction to the words.

- You're stressed out by the many things on your to-do list. Instead of getting overwhelmed, try saying to yourself, "I know

I can't do all of this at once, and I may not get to everything. I can be present in this moment and focus on the task at hand. By choosing to focus in the present, I'll feel calmer and be more efficient than if I obsess about all the tasks on my list."

- You're in a conversation and you find yourself having extraneous thoughts. Take a slow, full breath, and mindfully notice those other thoughts, and then let them go, bringing yourself back into your initial conversation.

- You're in the shower feeling anxious about a big presentation you need to make or a difficult conversation you need to have. Choose to take a minute for yourself to simply be aware of the sensation of warm water washing over your skin. You'll instantly feel more relaxed, and when you come back to thinking about the day ahead of you, you'll calmly come up with creative ways to articulate the points you want to make.

Unplug to Be Mindful

Unfortunately, our society praises us for multitasking. We all know we're not supposed to text and drive, but it turns out that talking on the phone while driving is just as dangerous. However, instead of enacting laws to prohibit this behavior, the world finds ways to enable it with hands-free devices.

Rudeness seems to now be an acceptable behavior as well. I've been at meetings where everyone attending had smartphones, laptops, or tablets on the conference table, and it was seen as completely acceptable to use them while other people were speaking.

Yet the reality is that when you try to do two things at the same time, you're not really doing either of them well. When you're multitasking, you're flitting back and forth between attention to one activity and then attention to the other, and so there will always be a sacrifice. So while it's "cool" right now to be totally "wired," in a couple of years I predict that people will realize they haven't really been paying attention. All of a sudden, that super new phone will lose its luster once you realize your needs aren't getting met or you're not meeting other people's needs because you're focused on something else all the time.

So before the rest of the culture catches up to us, we recommend starting the trend of being mindful. Unplug yourself for an hour a day. Turn yourself off. The truth is, our brains evolved in relation to nature, not to cell phones. If you can spend a part of your day in nature, you're going to feel profoundly different from when you're glued to your BlackBerry, Android, or iPhone.

The benefit will be that we become satisfied with less instead of excited to have more. In the same way, if you sit down to a meal and you're already full, you're not going to appreciate that meal very much. But if you're genuinely hungry, you can eat just one little thing, and it's going to be exquisitely satisfying.

Developing a More Spiritual Brain

The lessons in this chapter offer one way for us to tap into our spirituality. But as I said earlier, mediation and a spiritual life are not mutually exclusive: you can be a spiritual person and not meditate; and you can meditate without being a spiritual person. However, for people who are not in touch with their spirituality, meditation can provide the opportunity to step inside this unseen world.

At Canyon Ranch, we believe that spirituality is a critical component of brain health. My colleague and friend Dr. Allan Hamilton is a professor and neurosurgeon who believes that as a species, we have developed a spiritual or religious trait through natural selection. We know that the human brain is first and foremost a survival instrument. Hamilton believes that this particular characteristic of thinking or perception may have had a physical foundation: people who are spiritual have a psychological or emotional benefit that translates into a survival advantage. Someone who thinks the world is completely random and therefore has to deal with it as chance, without any ability to control or interpret what's happening, may be at a distinct disadvantage in terms of dealing with stress, as compared with someone who believes the world is a divine manifestation. Having a spiritual interpretation of the world helps us maneuver through it, understand it, and be more adept at explaining it.

Ultimately, we each live by mapping out our experience. Some of us are very practical and use a scientific map; others have an emotional map, an artistic map, and even a spiritual map. A Canyon Ranch we believe that when you learn to overlay these maps, you can create a balanced view of the world that leads to a fuller understanding of yourself and your health and ultimately can guide you toward happiness.

Incorporating spirituality into your everyday life can reduce stress and anxiety and can allow you to develop a more creative brain. When considering the spiritual quest, you have to imagine a whole different set of rules, and you will never know whether they exist or not. It allows you to think less rationally and more creatively about everything because if you can accept spirituality, it opens the door to accepting lots of other possibilities and choices for every aspect of your life. As one of the five pillars of peak performance, spirituality then becomes an opportunity to view your life in a completely different way, what we at Canyon Ranch like to call the Power of Possibilities.

PART THREE

Beyond Traditional Therapies

Chapter 9

IMPORTANT MEDICAL TESTING

If you've been following the thirty-day Canyon Ranch program of diet, exercise, and meditation, you may already be feeling better. Aside from its own positive benefits, each of these components allows you to start taking charge of your health, and just by doing so you may find that you are less anxious. You may be sleeping better as well, and this takes some of the stress off your brain. And by focusing on organic food choices, or possibly trying an elimination diet, you are beginning to remove the harmful toxins that may have been affecting your thinking.

Brain performance doesn't increase overnight. You'll be likely to experience incremental improvements that continue as long as you stick with the program. You may find that your brain fog lifts first, so you can think more clearly and make better decisions. As you master the aspects of the program that reduce stress, you'll be able to see clear enhancements of your memory and attention.

However, there are times when lifestyle changes aren't enough. If you follow this program for the full thirty days and do not see any improvement in your mood, thinking, or memory, it may be time to investigate your overall health. While you've already learned how your physical health affects your brain, this chapter outlines the discussions you can have with your doctor so that together you can diagnose and possibly reverse a deeper or distinct health issue.

BE A FAMILY DETECTIVE

You can begin to put together your own health profile by interviewing family members—your first-degree relatives, meaning your parents and siblings. These are the people who share your genetic information, so it's important to have a record of their symptoms, conditions, and illnesses. You can then bring this document to your doctors so that they can better understand your unique health situation.

Sometimes, obtaining this information is easier said than done. Some parents do not want to worry their children about their current or past health concerns and are unwilling to participate. If you were adopted, or lost a parent to illness or an accident, you might have limited data to work with, especially in terms of brain health. As you've learned, most signs of dementia do not become evident until individuals are in their later years.

At the same time, you need to look at the data you collect and decide how this information translates into your own life. Some of the information you come across may be behavioral in nature, and not a biological predisposition or risk factor. For example, if someone in your family died of a heart attack at age fifty, they might not have been predisposed to heart disease, but rather was a victim of addictive behavior. Or if someone died in a motorcycle accident, they might have been predisposed to risky behavior.

For More Information . . .

A good resource for creating a detailed family history, especially regarding your genetic blueprint, is the Surgeon General's Family History Project, available online. Visit www.familyhistory.hhs.gov to access the tools you'll need to work with your family.

Your own children can be another source of information. It's very common for parents who test a child for attention deficit disorder (ADD) to be surprised to find that they themselves test positive for ADD. This type of testing simply didn't exist before the 1970s, and many people's errant behaviors were written off as "rambunctiousness" or "scatteredness" when in fact they may have been suffering from a treatable illness.

GET THE BEST PHYSICAL POSSIBLE

A thorough medical history and a physical exam are the best ways to identify what aspect of your health is affecting your brain function. These include all the basics that your doctor typically performs, but it is important that you let him or her know that you are specifically concerned about your brain health. At Canyon Ranch, in order to meet our guests' needs, after a history and physical exam, we may use standard labs, biomarkers, and in some cases genetic testing to determine their current health status. A complete physical would emphasize blood pressure and pulse—both the rate and the rhythm—and examinations of the eyes, including the retina; heart and circulatory system; reflexes; strength; balance; coordination; and sensation. Your doctor may also investigate your skin and nails to determine if you have nutritional deficiencies.

The next level of questioning should involve ruling out potential diagnoses. For example, Parkinson's disease can present like Alzheimer's disease or dementia, but it is associated with other findings as well and needs to be treated correctly. In addition to showing symptoms of dementia, Parkinson's sufferers are stiffer, they shake, they have more difficulty with walking, and they lose their arm swing.

The most common cause of dementia that many doctors haven't considered is postoperative cognitive dysfunction. This can occur after a major operation involving general anesthesia, such as heart surgery, a hip replacement, or a knee replacement, and frequently occurs when the patient is over sixty-five years old. Many people complain that following a surgical procedure they start losing things, become uncomfortable driving due to changes in attention, or never get back to their previous level of functioning. While some might assume that these symptoms are a normal part of aging, the truth is that the brain has been negatively affected. It's important to discuss this issue with your doctor if you are experiencing symptoms and have had surgery, or if you are contemplating any sort of elective procedure that is accompanied by general anesthesia.

Other signs of some types of dementias actually occur during sleep. The second most common form of dementia is known as *Lewy body dementia,* and its earliest symptom is thrashing about in sleep, or kicking and screaming in the middle of the night. Many times a spouse is the first one to bring it to a doctor's attention. This can also be determined from a sleep study, as we discussed in chapter 5.

Important Medical Testing

Your doctor may suggest a series of blood tests to eliminate other medical issues. Blood tests can rule out an infection, cerebral vascular disease, diabetes, or a vitamin deficiency, all of which could be affecting your brain. Besides the tests that typically accompany a traditional physical and may show a correlation to poor brain health, like those for heart disease and diabetes, you may want to discuss with your doctor if it is reasonable to run additional tests. For example, a test for Lyme disease may be necessary if your history and physical suggested this could be a possibility. This tick-borne disease is growing in prevalence across the country and can affect the brain.

The C-reactive protein test is a very important measurement of how much inflammation is currently occurring in your body. As you've learned, increased inflammation could be affecting every aspect of your health, including your thinking, and needs to be reduced. The people who have the lowest levels of inflammation are also the most resistant to getting other infections or illnesses. For preventing or delaying Alzheimer's, you need to maintain a very low CRP. In a twenty-five-year prospective from the Honolulu-Asia Aging Study, researchers found that people with the lowest risk of Alzheimer's had the lowest CRP.

Genetic Testing

If you believe you have a medical history that puts you in the high-risk category for Alzheimer's disease, then genetic testing might be an appropriate option to discuss with your doctor. This type of testing identifies what your biological risk is relative to the population in general, for your gender—it allows people to get a sense of where they are in relationship to everybody else. Genetic testing can also be very useful if you were adopted and have limited data on or access to your birth parents.

In terms of Alzheimer's disease, currently the most important of the genetic tests is the ApoE4, because carrying this gene increases a person's risk of getting Alzheimer's by two to three times, compared with someone who does not have the gene. Having two of these genes raises your risk by twenty or thirty times.

It's important to understand that you are more than your genome. However, it is another bit of circumstantial evidence to support or lessen the likelihood of your having Alzheimer's disease and provides you with some direction as to what you can do now to prevent or delay the onset.

Identifying Toxins

When we test for toxins at Canyon Ranch, most people have an average of one hundred chemicals in their system. These tests are typically performed as hair, urine, or blood screenings. We usually perform these along with some genetic testing to see how good a detoxifier you are. We usually like to get the genetic facts to see which liver enzymes are weaker. One good test is referred to as liver genomics, and it gives us a report of what one's genetic propensity is in detoxifying various compounds that we produce internally, as well as external exposures.

TALK TO YOUR DOCTOR ABOUT THE FOLLOWING TESTS

Name of Test	What It Determines
C-reactive protein (CRP)	Inflammation: a marker for heart disease, stress, and general inflammation
Lyme panel	Lyme disease
ApoE4	Presence of genes related to Alzheimer's disease
Vitamin B_{12}	Vitamin B_{12} deficiency
HgbA1C and glucose tolerance test	Diabetes, insulin resistance
Blood, hair, urine toxicity screenings	The presence of heavy metals
Liver genomics	Liver's capacity to detoxify various compounds
Adrenal testing	Cortisol and DHEA; potential impact of stress on brain function
Plasma amino acids	Precursors to neurotransmitters
Omega-3 fatty acids	Levels of DHA
Hormone levels (thyroid, testosterone, estrogen, progesterone)	Hormone levels
Food sensitivity testing	Potential impact of immune response to food antigens and the impact on brain function
Celiac panel	Gluten sensitivity and its impact on depression

MEDICATIONS THAT AFFECT YOUR BRAIN

Some medications affect cognitive abilities, causing brain fog, increased fatigue, dizziness, and forgetfulness, and detract from focus and concentration. This is true of both prescription medications and over-the-counter remedies. What's more, combining prescription medications with over-the-counter remedies can also cause cognitive problems.

Some medications cause issues in the body that affect the brain. For example, Protonix and Prilosec, the proton pump inhibitors used for controlling stomach acid, can interfere with your ability to digest food. You need stomach acid to absorb Vitamin B_{12}, which is crucial for your brain. They also interfere with your ability to absorb some minerals, such as calcium, magnesium, and proteins, and when you don't have these nutrients in your blood, your brain cannot function well.

Antidepressants may have long-term effects on the brain. Antidepressants and other anxiety medications that normalize brain function may cause some degree of damage, including suicidal thoughts or nighttime binge eating. Even something as innocuous as Tylenol presents some risk. Studies have shown that people who take Tylenol often seem to have a higher chance of developing Alzheimer's. While it's a small increase in risk, it's significant.

The prescription medications on the following list can all affect your thinking. Speak to your doctor to determine if there are alternatives with fewer mental side effects. This is a very comprehensive list, but it is important to be very inclusive, as we really don't know how any one individual will be affected by a medication, let alone a combination.

Allergy medications
Amphetamines
Analgesics
Antibiotics
Anticholinergics
Antidepressants
Antidiarrheals
Antiepileptics
Antihistamines
Antihypertensives
Antipsychotics
Antiseizure medications
Anxiety medications

Barbiturates
Blood pressure medications
Blood sugar medications
Decongestants
Nausea medications
Pain medications
Parkinson's disease
    medications
Sedatives
Sleep medications
Stimulants
Tranquilizers
Ulcer medications

EVALUATE YOUR MEMORY

Your doctor may suggest that you take a mental assessment test. These tests establish your current cognitive abilities so you can create a baseline of information. With that you can then monitor any changes that occur, both positive and negative.

At Canyon Ranch we use two different types of assessments: the Wechsler Memory Scale, which is administered by a person; and MindStreams from NeuroTrax, which delivers testing online. Both tests assess cognitive function by measuring performance on a series of interactive tests and comparing the results with those of general population peer groups, based on age and education. Each determines your present capabilities in the following categories:

- Attention
- Executive function
- Information processing
- Memory
- Motor skills
- Verbal function
- Visual spatial perception

The next step is to obtain a diagnostic image of the brain to see if there are signs of damage, atrophy, stroke, or blood clot. The best type of scan currently available is the positron-emission tomography (PET) scan. The PET scan has the distinct advantage of being able to show areas of the brain that might have a problem before it would be detected on a CAT scan or MRI. For this reason, it is thought to be the best way to diagnose early Alzheimer's and early dementia.

PET scans are noninvasive, accurate, and fast. They detect disease on the cellular level by producing digital pictures and measuring the temperature functionality of different organs, including the brain. A PET scan works by using small amounts of a radioactive tracer, which chemically attaches to glucose in cells. As the glucose metabolizes it, the tracer emits radiation, which is detected by the scanner. The scanner records these signals and transforms them into images.

HAVE YOUR EYES CHECKED

We also suggest that you obtain a good eye examination. The eye is a window to the brain as well as being able to reveal changes that denote many systemic diseases; this is why a proper exam performed by an ophthalmologist offers another opportunity to discover dysfunction. An eye examination can reveal blood flow issues, certain cataracts, and even macular degeneration, which is linked with brain problems. We suspect that in the future, the eye exam will become the new way to diagnose brain problems like early Alzheimer's.

Chapter 10

SELECT COMPLEMENTARY
THERAPIES

The majority of this book has been written from the perspective of what many would call allopathic, or conventional Western, medicine. However, that is only one approach for maintaining and improving health, particularly when it comes to the brain. Many other effective therapies exist that have been used for hundreds, if not thousands, of years and developed in other parts of the world. Today, the most advanced doctors and researchers are uncovering the science behind many of these ancient techniques and are learning specific ways they can be incorporated into an approach that is referred to as *complementary medicine*, the blending of ancient practices and modern medicine to achieve the best results for treating or preventing illness and promoting health and well-being. In fact, members of our staff are at the forefront of this research.

At Canyon Ranch, we embrace complementary medicine; it's the underlying principle of how we treat our guests every single day. We believe that Western medicine and what many refer to as Eastern medicine can work side by side. What's more, we have found that some people respond to Eastern medical techniques when Western practices of medication or even surgery have not been fully effective.

Our integrative medicine experts have long recognized that many forms of hands-on—and hands-free—healing are safe and effective. Does that mean that every single disease should be treated by an Eastern medicine practitioner? The answer is no: when you have diseases that are easily definable, such as a bacterial infection, Western medicine can resolve the problem. But many times, an illness or symptom is a sign that the rest of the body, or the brain, is out of balance. That's when Eastern practices can be the most effective, especially when they are integrated with modern, Western notions of preventive therapies, such as diet and exercise.

The underlying principle of many of these therapies is that they treat the whole person. Let's face it, even when our stomach is bothering us, we're not just a stomach. We're not just an elbow. We're not just our nasal passages, or a brain. We're a whole being. Eastern therapies address the entire body by balancing and clearing our internal flow of subtle energy. This flow of energy is known as chi in China, as prana in India, and by other names in many other cultures.

Canyon Ranch has had a long-standing interest in energy and healing going back to its very inception. When Mel and Enid Zuckerman, the founders of Canyon Ranch, were first looking for a property, they came to what has become our Tucson resort and immediately felt the energy and the magic of the place. And over the years, the ranch has actually managed the largest sweep of energy and energy-related services of any facility in the country, if not the world.

Energy therapies may be effective for inducing relaxation, and as we know, when we can fully relax and let our anxieties dissipate, our cognitive function can increase. We do not wholly understand the mechanism through which energy therapies encourage the relaxation response, but it has been clearly shown that they do in some patients. The two therapies with the most scientific validation and the highest standards for practitioners are healing touch and acupuncture, both of which may improve brain health and are examples of complementary therapies.

ENERGY MEDICINE

Energy medicine is new to the scientific community, but it has been practiced for thousands of years. In the simplest terms, the experience of receiving energy healing is similar to massage, although you are not physically manipulated. People will typically report that they feel very relaxed, very peaceful after a session of energy healing: it reduces stress and anxiety, and for many, it reduces pain. These effects can lower blood pressure as well as improve mood, so it's not surprising that energy healing may affect brain health. And so, although the energy work might be on the hands or the head or the feet, that energy is ultimately going to affect the brain.

Energy healing techniques have also been used for people who have brain-related diseases or dysfunctions. Studies are currently being done using energy healing with people who have multiple sclerosis (MS), are recovering from concussions, or have brain trauma. And researchers are studying using energy healing to reduce distress in order to improve cognitive functioning for those with dementia.

HOW ENERGY MEDICINE MAY WORK

At Canyon Ranch we believe that science helps us to understand the invisible forces that surround us. We're learning more and more that there are things that our senses can't pick up, and what our senses detect is energy.

We've all heard of Einstein's famous physics equation: $E = mc^2$. Einstein proved that everything is made of energy, and energy can be converted into physical matter, and matter can be converted into energy. What we call matter is in actuality organized or crystallized energy. Although we experience the world as material, the world is not material. Everything that exists, whether it's called "inanimate" or "animate" from an energy point of view, is simply exchanging energy and information with its environment; no matter whether it's water molecules or DNA molecules or cells or a heart or the whole body, we're always receiving energy and information, and at the same time, we're expending energy and information.

Our bodies are made up of countless molecules that vibrate along with the energy fields that surround us, and all the complex systems of life that reside inside our bodies are regulated by streams of chemical and electrical messages. Every organ in the body is generating electrical signals, and the brain is no exception. It can communicate with every other organ in the body biochemically and electrically. So the brain is not just a material organ but an energy organ. It is receiving energy and emitting energy. The electrical impulses of the heart can be measured by an electrocardiogram (EKG) and those of the brain by an electroencephalogram (EEG). The heart's energy affects the brain's energy and plays a fundamental role in emotional and cognitive health. For optimal well-being, the entire body must be healthy and balanced.

We also know that when people touch or are in proximity to each other, there is an energy exchange. When one person lays hands on another, the two people are completing an electrical circuit. According to a 1994 study, one person's heartbeat signal is registered in another person's brain waves. This concept is the central scientific principle behind many healing techniques. While this signal is strongest when people are in physical contact, it is still detectable when subjects are near each other but not touching. What's more, the brain registers and can respond to another person's electrical signal, or energy. If the brain is registering changing electrical fields, then it's possible that it is biochemically changing. Research also shows that one person's brain can affect the electrical activity of another person's brain; this is true of people who are personally connected, such as friends or family members, and of healers working with patients.

We also believe that the energy from one person's heart can affect another. The human heart generates a powerful electromagnetic signal that can be directed to anyone including yourself whom you might want to help or whose pain, sadness, or illness you want to heal. This may be the elusive answer to the scientific question: "What exactly is love?"

For More Information . . .

For more information on the power of energy healing and energy body work, visit the Canyon Ranch website (www .canyonranch.com/energyheal ing) or download the Canyon Ranch "360 Well-Being" iPad app.

Energy healing practices therefore address restoration and achieving balance for the brain and the body. Professionally trained energy healers use nothing but their hands during hands-on healing and therapeutic touch. Practitioners channel ambient energy through their hands to the patient.

EXPLORING HEALING TOUCH AT HOME

Healing touch is a gentle, nurturing, entirely noninvasive energy practice in which practitioners gently hold areas of the body or hold their hands and inch or two away from the body. It has been shown to reduce anxiety, relieve stress and sleep disturbances, and help combat depression.

The following exercises can connect you with your own capabilities as an energy healer. If you can repeat these exercises regularly, you may feel more energized, calm, and clear. Give yourself at least fifteen minutes for each of the following exercises.

Exercise 1: Energy Practice

Sit comfortably with your hands, palms up, resting on your thighs. Invite the universal positive and healing energy that flows all around us and in us to enter your body. Visualize this energy passing from your brain, through your heart and body, and out your hands. Direct this peaceful healing energy to a person, an animal, or the whole world. Imagine this energy cycling in you, coming out of you, going to another person, and then coming back.

Exercise 2: Heart-Healing Energy

In this exercise you will be tapping into your heart's electromagnetic field as a source of healing. Afterward your brain and your body will feel energized and relaxed.

Place your left hand over your heart and your right hand over your upper abdomen. As you inhale, think "love heart" and think of drawing healing energy into your heart. As you exhale, think "love breath" and picture the energy pulse of your heart traveling to your lungs. Continue breathing and visualizing for several minutes.

If you are having pain or a disturbance in an area of your body (an upset stomach or a headache, for example) place your left hand as described above, and your right hand on the part of your body that is ailing, and continue the exercise.

Exercise 3: Stop Negative Energy

You can protect your brain from negative energy coming from the stressors in your life. This includes personal issues, poor health, and exposure to environmental toxins, as well as exposure to the electric waves from cell phones, computers, and other devices. You can use this simple, powerful exercise whenever you are feeling overwhelmed or overstressed and may experience the sensation of a cool mist as you practice it regularly.

Sit comfortably, and begin by inhaling slowly and deeply as you think the phrase "Protect brain." Visualize protective energy flowing up from the earth beneath your feet into your body, your heart, and your brain. When you exhale, think, "Protect out," and feel that powerful energy flow up from your heart and over your head, creating a showering shield of safety all around your body.

Acupuncture

Acupuncture is an ancient Chinese modality that has successfully been practiced for thousands of years and has been used by and studied in Western medicine—for example, at the National Institutes of Health. It is useful in addressing problems such as pain, arthritis, migraines, tension headaches, asthma, tendinitis, and fatigue, as well as enhancing immunity, decreasing anxiety, and treating insomnia. It is also used preventively as a tool for avoiding illness and promoting longevity.

Acupuncture is used to maximize energy and functioning throughout the brain and the body. In Chinese medicine, the body is thought to contain distinct internal pathways, or meridians. When these meridians become inactive, energy is blocked within the body, and health problems arise. Acupuncture moves what's known as chi, or a vital force, throughout your body and keeps the flow of energy going. When this happens, your body acts like a babbling brook, and you should feel relatively good. When the energy cannot move, you'll feel more like a stagnant swamp.

This ancient practice is thought to be useful in promoting overall brain health. The brain and body are first connected through the spinal cord, which joins the nerves of the brain to the nerves of the body. Acupuncture can be effective for the brain because it taps into nerves on the body, primarily in the hands and feet, that are linked to the brain via the central nervous system. For example, receiving an acupuncture treatment in a toe affects your brain because of the connection of the nerves of the toe to the spinal cord, which is connected to the brain. In China acupuncture continues to be used alongside Western medicine for a very large percentage of people who have neurological issues including stroke, dementia, and Parkinson's disease.

At Canyon Ranch, we have seen acupuncture help guests with depression improve focus and attention and clear brain fog. Usually when we feel unfocused, we're out of balance, and acupuncture is a quick way of getting back our balance. It provides a restorative sensation, similar to the way you feel after you've had a great night's sleep and you're ready to take on the day. Interestingly, the energy it provides actually helps the brain calm down, encouraging the body's own natural healing ability. We have found that when the body learns to fix itself, the results last.

Scientific studies of acupuncture all come to the same conclusion: when participants are given these therapies, they improve. However, why they improve remains a mystery. From a medical perspective, acupuncture seems to move the recipient out of the *sympathetic nervous state,* also known as the fight-or-flight response, and into a *parasympathetic state,* which is where the brain and the body can begin rebuilding, restoring, and relaxing. The relaxation includes your anxieties. That shift in states happens regardless of whether you are treating low-back pain, cancer, or dementia: it allows your body to almost immediately relearn how to relax, one reason why insomnia and other sleep issues are frequently treated with acupuncture.

Acupuncture treatments build on each other, and although they take time to produce results, many people experience profound change. Because acupuncture addresses a root imbalance instead of relieving specific symptoms, you may require anywhere from a few treatments to a few months of treatment. The longer you have had the problem, the more sessions you will probably need. The first signs that it is working include achieving a deep, refreshing sleep or a sense that you're happier and have a greater sense of well-being.

A Typical Visit to an Acupuncturist

A visit to an acupuncturist begins with a very thorough medical intake, including a health and personal history from early childhood up to the present. It is important that you feel comfortable with your practitioner and that you tell him or her about any conventional medications you are taking. Next you will receive tongue and pulse diagnoses. The practitioner will monitor nine pulses in each wrist and will be determining more than eight qualities in each pulse point. The tongue is important to the practitioner because different areas of the tongue relate to different organs in the body, and the cracks of the tongue and its coating are also key indicators of your health.

Once a diagnosis is made, a practitioner will insert very fine needles into the skin to produce the therapeutic effect. The idea that it will hurt to be stuck with needles keeps some people from considering acupuncture, but this is a misconception. The sterile needles used by qualified acupuncturists are much thinner than any needles used in conventional medicine—they are about the diameter of a human hair. The general amount of time the needles stay in the body is twenty to twenty-five minutes; it takes that long for the energy to circulate through the major meridians. There are, however, a few exceptions where slightly longer treatments may yield better results.

An interesting fact about acupuncture it that the needles are often not placed at the locations of the symptoms; for example, if you are having a problem with your left ankle, the needles might be placed on the right wrist or ankle so that the "healthier side," where more chi exists, can help out the less healthy side. When you begin to see an improvement, the practitioner may then needle the affected side. If the problem is chronic or low-grade, the practitioner may put the needles right in the area itself.

Almost any body part can be used to treat any other body part. The hands and feet contain more nerve endings than anywhere else, and in Chinese medicine, those areas are recognized as the location where all the meridians either begin or end. That is why they are considered to be the strongest points on the entire body and can be used to treat

Choosing the Right Acupuncturist

We recommend that you find a practitioner who is licensed by the National Certification Commission for Acupuncture and Oriental Medicine. Only a few states in the country don't license acupuncturists, including Wyoming, North Dakota, South Dakota, Kansas, Oklahoma, Louisiana, and Alabama. California and New Mexico have their own state accreditations that are even more rigorous than the national board exam.

almost any disease, including neurological problems. The traditional treatment for severe neurological problems, such as Parkinson's, stroke, and palsy, usually involves scalp acupuncture. The scalp is an acupuncture microsystem, as are the palms, soles of the feet, and ears.

Often, the first time people receive acupuncture they experience a tremendous change in their well-being. Some report a euphoric feeling, which may be due to a huge energy shift, especially if they started in a state of relative imbalance. Subsequently, it's actually a good sign if you don't experience this euphoric state after each session, because that means you're becoming more balanced, and therefore, you may not notice as dramatic a shift from the beginning to end of the treatment.

QIGONG AND TAI CHI

Two other energy therapies worth mentioning are the Chinese practices of qigong and tai chi. Qigong is the foundation of martial arts, and tai chi is a graceful and beautiful offshoot. Qigong defines the basic movements that channel energy and direct it to certain parts of your body. The basic tenets of qigong include the conservation of energy that allows you to become healthier, stronger, and wiser. A 2011 study from Scotland showed that even for those with dementia, qigong can help improve concentration, spatial awareness, and skilled movement as well as enhance confidence, relaxation, and social skills.

Think of qigong as an internal workout for your chi rather than your muscles. It's actually revitalizing your body and giving you more energy to work with, so either you could overpower someone in a martial arts sense, or you could self-heal or just feel calmer. It's also a form of meditation, but it's directed at building and refreshing energy rather than strictly calming the mind. Tai chi is also thought to offer a wealth of physical and mental benefits. According to the Mayo Clinic, tai chi's focus on movement and breathing creates a state of relaxation and calm, reducing stress, anxiety, and tension. It is also thought to relieve depression.

In a sense, qigong and tai chi are like giving yourself acupuncture without the needles. But the difference is, acupuncture is more accelerated; you can get a lot of benefit and sometimes see some pretty dramatic results in a short amount of time. With qigong and tai chi, you need to practice over a longer period of time to see a benefit.

The most basic qigong pose you can practice at home is called Hug a Tree, and it's just what it sounds like. Standing tall, raise your arms and imagine that you are encircling a large tree. People who have practiced for years can stand like this for an hour or two without batting an eye, focusing on their breath and moving their energy through the meridians. In the beginning, most people can hold this pose for only a few minutes.

Walking Backward:
A Chinese Medicine Beginner's Practice

The Chinese believe that walking backward helps your brain in much the same way we believe that there is benefit in training with your less dominant hand. Even today, you will see people walking backward all over China. They walk with purposeful intent through a park or on flat surfaces without looking behind them; you'll even see people walking backward down the street. They believe this practice helps an aging brain to stay young.

This firmly held belief that walking backward can help prevent degenerative brain disease is also put into practice in Japan and Korea. The idea is that there's never a point of no return: we can always improve, and there's always opportunity for the body and the brain to self-heal.

You can try this practice at home. For example, you can purposefully turn off the TV, but this time, get there by walking backward. You can also use it as a form of exercise when you are out for a stroll, and choose to do it either the entire time or a portion of the time. However, we recommend that if you already have poor balance or are considered to be frail, have a rail nearby or something to hold on to.

Chapter 11

———

CHALLENGE YOUR BRAIN

The latest advances in medical imaging have shown us that some cognitive as well as physical changes to the brain take place slowly, over many years, and begin much earlier than we think. We often miss the very first signs of cognitive dysfunction. Yet if we took a memory and/or attention test in our thirties, and then were retested as little as ten years later, our performance would be expected to decline. The typical age when these changes become noticeable and bothersome to us is generally around seventy. However, if you look at norms for cognitive testing, dysfunction can start occurring in your forties and fifties. Behavioral changes—including irritability, low mood, and depression—will very often follow.

One reason why there is a delay in the recognition of cognitive and behavioral changes is that we instinctively learn to compensate for minute losses of brainpower. Just as you may have realized that it's best to bend your knees when you pick something up if you are afraid you'll hurt your back, we adopt mental strategies for keeping up the appearance that we are thinking just as sharply as ever. These can be as simple as driving more slowly, making lists, or creating mnemonic devices to remember the names of the planets. In fact, throughout our schooling, we've been taught many different techniques that help us to remember, and we use them throughout our life. Even taking photographs at family events and on vacations is a way to help us keep memory strong.

These tricks work because they mirror how memory works through association. By using them, we fool ourselves into believing our thinking is just as fast as it was when we were younger.

But the truth is that it is not. Memory, attention, reaction time, problem solving, and visuospatial reasoning ability all weaken as we get older. Functional MRIs of young people and of old people as they try to solve a problem show that the older people are actually using more of their brain. This may occur because they have more experiences to draw upon to solve the problem. However, the older brain is not as well organized; younger brains do not have to use as much brainpower to solve the same problem.

It's also important to recognize that not all aspects of cognition decline with age. For instance, vocabulary performance is pretty much maintained throughout the life span. The words we learn early in life are deeply embedded. When you experience that "tip of the tongue" feeling of searching for a word or name, it's not because you've lost the words, it's just that it takes the brain longer to retrieve them.

What's more, there are plenty of people who are sharp as a tack in virtually every cognitive domain well into their seventies, eighties, and even their nineties. Our focus at Canyon Ranch is to help people to age optimally, and so we strive to replicate what those people at the far end of the curve are doing that enables them to function well. And as with everything you've learned so far, many of the lessons for preserving and enhancing cognitive function are in the lifestyle arena. This is why we strongly feel that there are many things you can do right now to keep your brain sharp as you age. What's more, the earlier you start, the better your results will be: enhancing brain function now, before symptoms occur, will offer you the greatest protection well into your later years.

The secret, again, is neurogenesis, and in the case of maintaining a vibrant and actively thinking brain, the goal is twofold: to continue to create new synaptic connections by linking into existing brain cells, and to create new brain cells. As we've already discussed, this rewiring, referred to as neuroplasticity, is the brain's ability to change and grow as we learn new things, which assists in preserving cognitive function.

This chapter will discuss the areas within cognitive functioning that change as you age, and the ways you can begin to enhance them.

The Theory of Cognitive Reserve

Studies have proven that generally, people with a higher education have fewer end-of-life cognitive problems, yet we don't know why this is so. Some believe that well-educated people simply take better care of themselves and have better access to high-quality medical attention. Others believe, as we do, that a lifetime of learning is what gives you the mental horsepower to keep your brain strong. This concept is known as the *cognitive reserve theory*.

In 1988, a study published in *Annals of Neurology* revealed that upon autopsy some brains displayed extensive Alzheimer's disease damage, yet during their lifetime, those individuals had very few if any manifestations of the disease. The study also showed that these people had higher brain weights and a greater number of neurons as compared with other people of the same age group. The researchers determined that those with larger brains that held more neurons and neuronal connections may have had a greater "reserve" that protected them from developing cognitive symptoms of the Alzheimer's disease that was in fact present in their brains.

This theory suggests that ongoing educational and social life experiences may help develop a larger prefrontal cortex by activating neuroplasticity, helping you strengthen and grow neuronal connections and develop more efficient cognitive networks. A second longitudinal study confirmed these findings. In the Rush University Medical Center Religious Orders Study of 2004, it was found that over a five-year period, the participants who were more engaged with learning were about half as likely to develop Alzheimer's disease later in life.

On the basis of these findings, we at Canyon Ranch believe that continuous learning will allow you to avoid or reverse cognitive impairment in two distinct ways. First, you will make more neuronal connections as you learn (again, neuroplasticity). This benefits the brain as you age: when some of the older neuronal connections go bad, you'll have access to other ones. Second, these additional neuronal connections provide the brain with choice and opportunity; with more connections, you'll be able to devise alternative strategies or methods for solving problems, maintaining attention, and even accessing memory.

You may have built up some level of cognitive reserve already because of your IQ, your education, your occupation, and the leisure activities you choose, especially those that involve interaction with others. Yet these same attributes may mask early cognitive changes. If you have a high IQ, the way others perceive you, or even your scores on memory tests, may continue to be normal even though you've already begun to experience mild or moderate cognitive decline. It's like having the mental equivalent of $4 million in net worth. If you lose half of that, you're down to $2 million. Well, $2 million is still more than what most households in the Unites States have, and you may be able to continue to live your life successfully, and because of that you might not be motivated to improve or enhance your brain. But if you know that you used to have $4 million and you're down to $2 million, it might be the motivation you need to make these kinds of changes.

Another observation we've gleaned from testing hundreds of people at Canyon Ranch is that many very bright people are troubled by memory difficulties, but then discover when they are tested that, though they have noticed a real decline from their previous level, their memory is still way above average or even superior to that of others their age. This doesn't mean that you have to settle for even average test results, and you can't always rely on your cognitive reserve. There's always room to improve and reverse memory impairments, no matter where you are on the testing ladder.

COGNITIVE RESERVE IMPROVES EXECUTIVE FUNCTION

Cognitive functioning can be measured in a variety of areas. The first is straight performance, which involves testing that measures either attention or memory. If you participate in these types of tests, you would be asked to practice task A, and then later measure your performance on task A to see if you've improved. The results then are generalized to quantify your cognitive capacity, but in reality they measure only one type of task—the results are not applicable to entire brain function.

A better test is one that quantifies *executive function,* the brain's decision-making and goal-directed behaviors. In this scenario, you are trained on task A, and your results are tested in task A, but also on tasks B, C, and D. These tests can translate into success in real life because they cross domains. And because of this, we know that making connections between disparate topics, or simply continuing to make good decisions, is the real hallmark of a vibrant and active brain.

The Truth About Attention

Attention errors come in two distinct varieties: errors of *commission* and errors of *omission.* The first group refers to judgment mistakes. For example, an error of commission occurs when you are driving down a street and perceive that the car coming in the opposite direction is barreling right at you, forcing you to swerve to avoid it, only to realize there was plenty of room between the two cars. Another commission error could include hearing something other than what was actually said, or remembering that someone was present at a meeting when he or she was not really in attendance.

The more common mistake is an error of omission, which involves the absence of attention. A good example is when you don't see a car coming right toward you. This occurs because as we get older, we tend to focus on a narrower field of vision—the scope of our view becomes smaller, allowing for more missed events even when we are right in their midst. For example, the most likely traffic accident among older adults occurs during the making of a left turn, because drivers misjudge or don't see the oncoming traffic. Another common omission error could include forgetting that someone was at a meeting when he or she was actually present. This is also known as *selective attention.*

One of the best examples of errors of omission is a video created by former Harvard students Christopher Chabris and Daniel Simons. In it, a group of people are passing a basketball back and forth. There are three people with black shirts, three people with white shirts, and two basketballs. The people in black shirts pass only to others with black shirts. The people with white shirts pass only to others with white shirts. As the viewer, you are asked to count how many times the people with the white shirts pass the basketball. During the video, all the participants are moving around a circle in a small space. Then a person in a gorilla suit walks into the center of the circle and walks out. The gorilla is on the screen for 50 percent of the video, and the players have to accommodate their passing around the gorilla. After the video is over, you are asked to record how many times the basketball was passed. What's interesting is that 80 percent of the people who are shown the video don't see the gorilla at all.

This exercise is one of many that show that attention is actually a very limited resource. Unfortunately, unless we develop better attention skills, it is very likely that ours will only get worse as we get older. The aging brain is partly at fault: as the nervous system slows down as we get older, we have trouble doing each task well. But the bigger culprit in destroying our attention is our penchant for multitasking. Because we are constantly being challenged to keep up with our very hectic lives, our ability to limit our attention to one task goes down; this is why the idea of multitasking well is a myth. Talking on a cell phone while driving with perfect attention is just not possible.

If you want to improve your attention, you must practice clearing your mind of distractions and concentrate on one activity at a time. If you find yourself sidetracked by intrusive thoughts or other stimuli, you can develop the ability to let go of the distractions and effectively bring your attention back to the task at hand. Many of the quick meditation techniques from chapter 8 will help you increase your capacity to focus your attention.

See for Yourself

To see the selective attention test mentioned above, go to: www.youtube.com/ watch?v=vJG698U2Mvo.

Other exercises described later in this chapter can help you increase your field of vision.

Focus on the Right Kind of Learning

In order to build more cognitive reserve, not just any learning will do. When we look at the longitudinal studies, we observe certain characteristics in people who maintain well-preserved cognitive function into their later years. These people tend to seek out new experiences and learn how to do new things. They travel, they're curious, and they're interested in the world outside their communities. These types of new education are the exact recipe for making new neuronal connections as neuroplasticity.

Learning doesn't mean only acquiring new information; it also includes gaining new skills. In fact, discovering how to do something is actually more important than learning new information. While memorizing facts and philosophies will challenge your brain, acquiring a new skill is more effective for making new neuronal connections. New skills might include a new computer program, a new dance step, a new kind of exercise, a new craft activity, or a new game. You don't have to become an ultramaster at these new skills; it's the process that makes the greatest impact.

What's more, you need to constantly engage in this new learning, focusing on skills that get more difficult as you progress and become more proficient. It's just like exercise: if you simply want to stay in shape and your goal is to maintain your weight, you can do the twenty minutes of cardiovascular activity a day that most doctors recommend. But if you want to see real change, you're going to have to work harder.

Very few of us are engaged in education at the level that makes a difference in maintaining and enhancing brain health. Worse, there's a whole cottage industry of books, brain games, and other activities that are supposed to make us smarter or think faster but that really don't work. The biggest waste of time is rote memorization or convoluted memory tricks. Memorizing bits and pieces of information doesn't have a correlation to improving executive function, even though it comes in handy when you want to impress your friends or play trivia games.

We once had a guest at Canyon Ranch who was a math professor on a national trivia team, and we were all pretty impressed with what he knew: he could recite the value of pi to twenty-eight decimal places. He remembered the first four digits were the same as the year of the Battle of Agincourt, and the next four digits meant something else to him, and so on. But even though he "knew" so much, his executive function scores were low.

For the same reason, crossword puzzles may be less effective in increasing neuroplasticity. Crossword puzzles also have a certain element of memorization of trivia, so you're not really making new connections. Worse, there are a finite number of two-letter words and other spelling oddities, and crossword puzzle makers and solvers tend to learn those tricks. Some people will do crossword puzzles from just one resource or in one specific domain (such as celebrity weddings), so they are again stuck learning the same trivia. And lots of people focus on the puzzles they know they can do, instead of stretching themselves to work out the tough ones. Again, without the strain, you've lost the benefit.

Other games and activities, even in math and the sciences, that don't get progressively harder are not going to cause positive neuroplasticity. Sudoku is probably not going to change the structure of your brain. Social card games like bridge aren't going to do it, either, unless you are concentrating intently, remembering which cards

Curiosity Is a Brain Workout

Another way to keep your mind from aging is to continuously look for new challenges. We all have a natural tendency toward curiosity, so take advantage of this drive to learn. While developing new skills is most important, using your curiosity to seek out those skills is critical. It's just like exercise. While we know that aerobic exercise is the best for brain health, you still need to stretch, because it will help you to be better at your aerobic exercise. Your curiosity will take you to the skill that will interest you most.

have been played, and thinking flexibly about which cards to play next. However, competition seems to be a factor: the motivation to win can make you work harder at playing a game, and you'll learn more.

Be Social

There is also a social component in postponing the aging of the brain. As we discussed earlier, people who are more socially engaged tend to stay cognitively healthy. We suggest that you look for activities you can do that combine elements of high socialization and speed. When you can practice new skills with others, this helps to create an optimal brain-challenging environment. For best brain enhancement, choose activities that require learning a new skill, such as dance, or playing board games or doing other activities where you could add a speed component. One good example is playing Scrabble with a time limit, where you have to make your move in thirty seconds. So while chess and backgammon are acceptable choices, better ones would be the speedier versions. Playing charades is another way to combine these two attributes and engage your brain at the same time.

Learn a Second Language

Knowing a second language is a terrific way to establish cognitive reserve, and learning a second language later in life helps to create more of it. In one Canadian study, participants who were bilingual from very early ages were monitored and were found to have an average age of the onset of dementia that was four years later than that of speakers of only one language. At Canyon Ranch we believe that secondary language fluency has a great protective effect because it is a new skill and is even more effective when it has a tangible, personal meaning. For example, if you're planning to travel to France, and you're really excited about it, you'll actively engage in learning to speak French, which would then make a greater difference to your brain health.

Learning a second language is better for the brain because you can't fake your success. Typically, people can compensate their way around most casual conversations in their native tongue, even if they don't know anything about the topic at hand. They can express an opinion in generalities, and logically think their way through it. However, mastering a second language has a nice quantifiable aspect: either you can speak it or you cannot. You can read it or you cannot. Best of all, you can begin to improve your brain simply by starting to learn new vocabulary in that language. You don't necessarily have to become fluent in order to reap all the benefits.

Computer Games

There has been a lot of controversial research about the effect computer games and our ubiquitous digital lifestyle have on the brain. Studies have shown that the more time we spend on computers and using smartphones, the more distracted we've become. In one study from German Sport University Cologne, playing video games led to markedly lower sleep quality than watching TV, and also led to a "significant decline" in the ability to remember vocabulary. Other studies have shown correlations between video games and poor mood. According to the *New York Times*, new research on children suggests a correlation between heavy gamers and depression.

But not all of the news is bad. Many games have been created for the sole purpose of increasing memory and attention, and some of them are quite good. One company we are particularly interested in is Posit Science. Its research documents that people who use its programs reverse their brain age by up to ten years. One reason the games are so effective is that they increase in difficulty, and their results are quantifiable. Even games on handheld devices, such as Nintendo's Brain Age, can help improve your cognitive performance. As with the Posit Science programs, the scores are quantifiable and the level of difficulty increases with use.

Driving video games are thought to be beneficial because they improve attention. This is because they are happening in real time, and you have to stay focused. Other games that can improve your field of vision and increase attention are those in which the player is required to keep track of many items on a screen at once. Both field-of-vision and driving games get progressively more difficult as they get faster and there are more things to keep track of. Studies have shown that these types of video games can improve driving skills, which means there is a real-world consequence. In one 2008 study funded by Allstate Insurance, researchers found that drivers who played these games were able to react more quickly because their field of vision had improved, along with cognitive ability. This is particularly significant because driving is integral to staying active and engaged in society. In another study, published in 2009 in the *Journal of Gerontology,* older drivers who completed speed-of-processing training were 40 percent less likely to stop driving over the subsequent three-year period; 14 percent of older drivers who did not receive speed-of-processing training were forced to stop driving; and only 9 percent of those who completed eight or more sessions of speed-of-processing training ceased driving.

All kinds of cognitive benefits come from doing the Posit Science program. The Posit Science folks have also found that when people do the program, their mood improves. So engaging in this cognitive-enhancement exercise for five hours a week over eight weeks helped people to improve their mood. That's because people know they're doing something good for themselves and taking care of their brain, and they feel empowered. When you have the feeling that "I'm getting smarter just doing this," it will enhance your mood.

There's also the buzz you get from completing the tasks. I've noticed that after an hour of doing them, I feel as if I've had a double espresso. If you are suffering from low mood or depression, the adrenaline rush that comes with successfully completing the game will improve your mood, an experience similar to the dopamine reward. Computer games may be designed to activate the dopamine pathway.

The combination of the actual stimulation of doing the exercise plus the good feeling about yourself that you get will enhance your improvement even further.

Musical Instruments

Music affects the brain on many different levels. Listening to relaxing music promotes better sleep and can improve mood, two key factors in advancing brain health. Some researchers also believe in the Mozart effect—the idea that learning how to play music can actually make you smarter—although subsequent studies have not supported this hypothesis.

Music recognition is distributed widely throughout the brain. The left hemisphere targets successions of sounds and rhythm, while the right hemisphere contains many other, more specific music areas. People who learn to play an instrument, or even to sing, exercise strong connections between these two hemispheres; such exercise increases cognitive capacity and trains the brain to be better organized. In other words, people who study music may be able to think more quickly and accurately, and develop increased memory capacity.

Learning to play an instrument also has the requisite quantifiable aspect. Much like learning a second language, your guitar playing is getting better or it's not. And if you find the process enjoyable, the benefits will be even greater.

Reading

Pleasure reading alone is not enough of a challenge to make permanent changes in the brain. Instead, focus on reading—either fiction or non-fiction—as if you were going to be tested on the material. You have to think about what you read as if you were preparing for a college-level class. So if you've always been interested in the history of the American Revolution, find a local adult-education university or community-college class that covers this era, and join in. In this way, you'll be reading at a higher level and engaging with others at the same time.

ENHANCING INTELLIGENCE

Cognition and intelligence are separate yet related factors of brain health. In order to increase intelligence, you have to be able to improve your brain speed to access your memories quickly and make new intellectual connections through the executive function. You also need to be able to focus your attention on incoming information in order to synthesize it into new memories.

Intelligence doesn't refer only to how smart you are, or how much trivia you know. There are many types of intelligence, and your levels of each fluctuate as you get older. It's quite common for people to be highly developed in one area and deficient in another. It's also very possible to improve all aspects of intelligence now and as you get older. In fact, the key to a high-functioning brain is to be able to enhance all domains of learning, and therefore all domains of intelligence.

Abstract IQ

Abstract IQ is perhaps the best-known. The typical Mensa genius has a high abstract IQ because he or she is able to synthesize facts, recognize patterns, and create new paradigms. Abstract IQ is the sum of the stuff you know and the information you can share with others, combined with your ability to manipulate your fund of knowledge. For most people, this is how they perceive how smart they are.

In order to enhance abstract IQ, you need to increase your fund of knowledge as well as engage in the logical recognition of patterns, problem solving, and the creation of new ideas. The fastest way to do this is to increase your opportunities for education. Reading the newspaper every day is a good start. However, most newspapers, even the national heavyweights, are written at only a sixth- to eighth-grade reading level. What's more, because they rush to print content daily, they are not always accurate in presenting the information they've gathered. If you get your information from only this type of source, you are not training your brain to think at a very high level. The weekly newsmagazines may be better because they have a week deadline and therefore more time to be more accurate and are written at a slightly higher reading level. But to see dramatic changes, you need to study as if you were taking a college course. This might include attending lectures in your area or following a curriculum that you can buy from businesses like the Teaching Company.

For More Information . . .

The Teaching Company's lecture series called The Great Courses is a terrific way to start enhancing brain function right at home. This company has recorded over 350 engaging professors on DVDs, audio CDs, and other formats. Since 1990, teachers from the Ivy League, Stanford, Georgetown, and other leading colleges and universities have crafted courses ranging through science, history, the arts, literature, religion, philosophy, business, and economics for individual sale. In order to get the most out of the experience, trade courses with family members or friends so you can engage in lively conversation and share what you have learned. For more information, go to www.thegreatcourses.com.

Creative IQ

Creative IQ is the ability to incorporate new ideas into established ways of doing things, leading to a change in viewpoint. Individuals with high creative IQs are often highly empathetic because they can see multiple points of view.

While some people are inherently more creative than others, many people have a greater capacity for creative thinking than they are actually using. For instance, certain types of educational environments and work settings encourage creative thinking, and other environments discourage it. There are many approaches to enhancing creative thinking that are used in educational and corporate settings to stimulate innovation and improve organizational effectiveness. Many of these methods teach individuals how to approach problems and situations from different perspectives. One we're fond of at Canyon Ranch is playing with toys or puzzles that require manual manipulation. These can be as complex as a Rubik's cube or as simple as a box of Legos. Especially for adults, these types of toys continue to unlock reasoning and assist in activating the parts of the brain required for creativity.

Emotional IQ

Emotional IQ (EQ) was first brought to public awareness by the author Daniel Goleman and includes being sensitive to others and being able to sustain relationships. The ability to see other points of view, and be empathetic toward others, is a large component of emotional intelligence. It also involves being aware of your own emotions and being able to handle them effectively. Emotional intelligence also relates to knowing what makes you happy, knowing how to successfully handle stress and negative emotions, and learning how to handle change and be resilient.

Emotional intelligence is just as fluid and flexible as other types; through learning and training you can change your personality in just the same way that you can become smarter. In order to increase emotional intelligence, you have to learn better ways of dealing with people. Any relationship in which you can learn about and appreciate other people's feelings and points of view can enhance empathy. This can happen in a good friendship or intimate relationship and often occurs in counseling and psychotherapy and in certain mentoring and coaching relationships. There are also self-help programs with specific exercises to enhance the capacity to consider other people's points of view.

One way to increase your emotional intelligence is through your exposure to different cultures. There's a world of difference between ethnic groups right in your own community. If you can share your customs and practices, others will share theirs, and you can develop a better understanding of other people. It's also important to understand how people of different income levels live. It's one thing to donate money to a community food bank, but a better way of understanding the people it serves would be to volunteer there. The more you can get outside your world, the more you will increase your emotional intelligence in many different ways.

In fact, volunteering your time is one of the best ways to preserve and enhance an aging brain. Michelle Carlson, PhD, the associate director of the Center on Aging and Health at Johns Hopkins Bloomberg School of Public Health, ran a study called the Experience Corps trial, in which older men and women volunteered to teach reading skills to kindergarteners through third graders in Baltimore city schools. In 2008, using brain-imaging studies, Carlson and her colleagues showed that after just a few months, people who volunteered displayed beneficial changes in their brains similar to those that other research teams have seen with exercise.

It may be that volunteering combines the best attributes of all these mental brain games: It requires new learning, because you are placed in a new situation with new people. It requires that you convey the mastery of a skill set. It is social and positively engaging. And last, it teaches empathy for others.

More Information, More Opportunities

Another opportunity for lifelong learning can be found with a MOOC: massive open online course. Many of the top universities around the world offer free classes in a wide variety of subjects through three primary vendors: Coursera (www.coursera.org), edX (www.edx.org), and Udacity (www.udacity.com). The classes are given as lectures, and many require outside work beyond watching the Internet videos in order to receive a certificate of completion. While you can dabble in many of these classes, remember that simply watching the videos won't enhance brain health; it's completing the assignments and synthesizing the new information that's going to make the greatest difference.

QUICK MEMORY TIPS

Enhancing memory does not lead to enhancing intelligence. However, there are times when you need to remember things—computer passwords, combination locks, birthdays, anniversaries, and more. This is when the time-tested memory devices come into play. They won't increase your brain health, but they will keep you out of trouble.

Next time you need to make sure information is stored in your brain so you can retrieve it, try any of the following:

- *Create a very short story.* Put the information inside a sentence. For example, memorize a password by creating a story around it, or connect it to another memory that is easy to recall. If your password was 7, 14, 22. Your story could be: "Seven sisters bought fourteen pairs of shoes, each costing twenty-two dollars."

- *Create a word or acronym.* If you have to memorize a list of items (such as a shopping list), place them in order so that the first letters create a new word. One example: TOAST, representing tomatoes, onions, apples, spinach, and turnips. Another favorite is the colors of the rainbow: ROY-G-BIV (red, orange, yellow, green, blue, indigo, violet).

- *Associate it with an image or an emotion.* Create a picture in your mind of whatever you need to memorize. For example, using the same password—7, 14, 22—you can think of a house with seven windows, fourteen flowers, and twenty-two steps to the front door. You can also attach a positive emotion to this house: imagine it's the one you've always dreamed of living in.

- *Limit distractions during learning.* When you try to memorize information, turn off as much of the outside world as possible. Go into a quiet space that is free from distractions and take a deep breath before using any of these suggestions. This will allow you to focus more intently, so that your brain can work harder at the one task of remembering, instead of parsing out all the background noises of life.

Chapter 12

BRAIN HEALTH RECIPES

As you've learned, there are many terrific foods that support brain health. Your next challenge is to put them together to create delicious meals your whole family will enjoy. At Canyon Ranch, our team of expert chefs uses these ingredients every day to prepare interesting and tasty meals for our guests. Now you can prepare the same meals right in your own home.

What follows are some of our favorite new recipes that support brain health. Each one highlights the nutrients discussed in Chapter 6 so you can clearly see the link between the foods you eat and improving brain health. We've also included traditional nutrition information for every recipe. Remember, this particular program is not about counting calories; that's simply not the Canyon Ranch way. However, you can use the nutritional information to see how each of these foods adds to your intake of macronutrients (protein, carbohydrates, and healthy fats) so you can balance your day.

The recipes are for a wide variety of serving sizes, as we've found that many are perfect for entertaining large and small groups. You can scale up the quantities as needed by multiplying. And if you enjoy these, check out our website at www.canyonranch.com/recipes, where we list dozens of wonderful recipes, many of which support brain health.

The Recipes

Breakfast

SUPER ANTIOXIDANT BLUEBERRY SMOOTHIE

Makes one 16-ounce smoothie

This smoothie is high in fiber and the micronutrients that combat oxidative stress. It's also dairy free, which means it's low-fat.

INGREDIENTS

1 cup blueberries
1 cup orange juice
Pinch ground cinnamon

DIRECTIONS

Combine all ingredients in a blender and blend until smooth.

NUTRITION INFORMATION PER SERVING

180 calories

42 g carbohydrate

2 g fat

0 mg cholesterol

2 g protein

4 mg sodium

4 g fiber

TROPICAL GRANOLA

Makes twelve ½-cup servings

This recipe is perfect for making a large batch ahead of time and using as needed. Divide the granola into individual zipper bags to keep fresh and to keep portion sizes accurate. For a complete breakfast, add vanilla yogurt and fresh berries to this granola to make a parfait. Feel free to substitute almond butter or peanut butter for cashew butter. If you can't find oat flour, you can use regular or quick rolled oats and grind them in a blender.

This granola is naturally a good source of protein, but will be a better protein meal when combined with yogurt. The oats, fruit, and nuts make this granola high in fiber and B vitamins, which support brain health. Its fiber content also slows the rate of glucose absorption and helps stabilize blood-sugar levels for several hours after eating, providing energy and appetite control.

INGREDIENTS

Canola oil spray
1½ cups rolled oats
½ cup oat flour
½ cup toasted coconut flakes
½ cup macadamia nuts
Pinch ground cinnamon
Pinch ground nutmeg
Pinch sea salt
2 tablespoons orange juice
    concentrate
1 tablespoon pineapple
    concentrate
¼ cup light coconut milk
1 tablespoon brown sugar
1 tablespoon pure vanilla extract
¾ teaspoon cashew butter
1 tablespoon pure maple syrup
½ cup dried pineapple, chopped
½ cup dried mango, chopped
2 tablespoons honey, heated

DIRECTIONS

1. Preheat oven to 275°F. Lightly spray a baking sheet with canola oil.

2. In a medium bowl, combine oats, oat flour, coconut flakes,

macadamia nuts, cinnamon, nutmeg, and salt and mix well. In a small bowl, combine orange juice concentrate, pineapple juice concentrate, coconut milk, brown sugar, vanilla extract, cashew butter, and maple syrup and mix well. Add to dry mixture and mix until moist.

3. Crumble mixture onto baking sheet and bake for 45 minutes to 1 hour, stirring after 25 minutes to allow for even cooking. Remove granola from oven, break apart while still slightly warm, and toss with dried fruit and honey. Cool on baking sheet.

NUTRITION INFORMATION PER SERVING
205 calories
34 g carbohydrate
5 g fat
0 mg cholesterol
7 g protein
52 mg sodium
4 g fiber

FRITTATA WITH SPINACH AND TOMATOES

Makes 8 servings

Eggs are an easy way to get protein into your breakfast routine, to help support critical thinking all day long. This recipe makes a delicious high-protein meal for the whole family in just one dish.

INGREDIENTS

Canola oil spray
8 large eggs
2 cups egg whites
¼ cup 2% (low-fat) milk
½ teaspoon fresh lemon juice
⅛ teaspoon extra virgin olive oil

1 cup tomatoes, diced
1 cup fresh spinach, chopped
¼ teaspoon sea salt
⅛ teaspoon freshly ground black pepper
1 cup shredded cheddar cheese

DIRECTIONS

1. Preheat oven to 375°F. Lightly spray a 9-inch cake pan with canola spray and set aside.

2. In a large bowl, whisk together eggs, egg whites, milk, and lemon juice.

3. Heat olive oil in a large sauté pan over medium-high heat. Sauté tomatoes and spinach briefly and season with salt and pepper.

4. Stir cheese and sautéed vegetables into egg mixture and pour into cake pan.

5. Bake frittata in oven until eggs are cooked and cheese is melted, about 20 to 30 minutes.

6. Remove from oven, let cool briefly, and cut into 8 pieces before serving.

NUTRITION INFORMATION PER SERVING

180 calories

7 g carbohydrate

7 g fat

219 mg cholesterol

20 g protein

420 mg sodium

1 g fiber

Lunch

FENNEL, ARUGULA, AND BLUEBERRY SALAD

Makes four 1-cup portions

This quick and easy salad is perfect to make for yourself or whenever you are entertaining. The blueberries are an interesting and unexpected addition, and they support brain health because they are high in fiber and antioxidants. This is also a sneaky way to get in another daily serving of fruit.

INGREDIENTS

For the French Vinaigrette

2 tablespoons garlic, minced

½ cup champagne vinegar or
    white wine vinegar

¼ cup Dijon mustard

3 tablespoons water

2 tablespoons low-sodium
    tamari sauce

¼ teaspoon freshly ground black
    pepper

2 tablespoons canola oil

2 tablespoons extra virgin olive
    oil

For the Salad

2 cups fresh fennel, shaved

1 cup arugula

1 cup fresh blueberries

DIRECTIONS

1. Place garlic in a strainer and submerge in a small pan of boiling water for 5 seconds or until garlic turns white.

2. Place garlic, vinegar, mustard, water, tamari sauce, and black pepper in a blender and puree until smooth. Slowly drizzle in canola oil and olive oil while blender is running and continue pureeing until well mixed.

3. In a large salad bowl, combine fennel, arugula, and blueberries; toss with the dressing; and serve.

NUTRITION INFORMATION PER SERVING
80 calories
11 g carbohydrate
3 g fat
0 mg cholesterol
1 g protein
147 mg sodium
3 g fiber

QUINOA AND WHITE BEAN SOUP

Makes eight 6-ounce servings

Soup is a great lunch because it fills you up but contains very few calories. This one is particularly satisfying because of the quinoa. This whole grain actually counts as a protein but feels like rice, making this soup an ideal way to support brain health by getting a full serving of vegetables and protein with very little fat.

Don't be afraid to open a can of beans and use only a little. You can store the remaining cannellini beans in an airtight container in the freezer for up to two months.

INGREDIENTS

1 tablespoon extra virgin olive oil

1 cup yellow onion, diced

¾ cup carrots, diced

¼ cup celery, diced

¼ cup fresh fennel, diced

One 14.5-ounce can no-salt-added diced tomatoes

4 cups vegetable stock

½ teaspoon dried basil

½ teaspoon dried oregano

¼ teaspoon dried marjoram

¼ teaspoon freshly ground
pepper

1¼ teaspoons sea salt

½ teaspoon Worcestershire
sauce

1 teaspoon low-sodium tamari
sauce

¼ cup quinoa

¼ cup canned cannellini beans,
drained

DIRECTIONS

1. Heat olive oil in a large stockpot over medium-high heat and add onion, carrots, celery, and fennel and cook until tender, about 5 minutes.

2. Add tomatoes, stock, herbs, pepper, salt, and Worcestershire and tamari sauces. Stir in quinoa. Bring to a boil and reduce heat to low. Cover and cook until quinoa pops open, about 20 to 25 minutes.

3. Stir in cannellini beans and let cook for another 5 minutes. Ladle ¾ cup soup into each bowl and serve.

NUTRITION INFORMATION PER SERVING

75 calories

11 g carbohydrate

2 g fat

0 mg cholesterol

2 g protein

272 mg sodium

2 g fiber

SALAD WITH SALMON BURGER AND GRILLED PINEAPPLE SALSA

Makes 4 servings

This is a perfect summertime salad that you can make on the grill or broil in the oven. Salmon is high in protein and important omega-3 fatty acids, which are critical to supporting brain health.

INGREDIENTS

For the Wasabi Salad Dressing

½ tablespoon horseradish

2 tablespoons canola mayonnaise

½ teaspoon wasabi powder

½ teaspoon Dijon mustard

⅓ cup low-fat sour cream

¼ teaspoon fresh lemon juice

¼ teaspoon sea salt

¼ teaspoon freshly ground black pepper

For the Salmon

1 pound fresh salmon, cut into 1-inch pieces

2 tablespoons low-sodium tamari sauce

1½ tablespoons tapioca starch

¼ teaspoon freshly ground black pepper

For the Salsa

Canola spray

1 pound fresh pineapple, peeled, cored, and sliced

¼ cup red bell pepper, diced

1 tablespoon red onion, diced

1 tablespoon scallions, chopped

1 tablespoon honey

2 teaspoons fresh lime juice

2 teaspoons ground cumin

1 tablespoon garlic, minced

1 tablespoon fresh cilantro, chopped

¼ teaspoon sea salt

2 cups mixed greens

DIRECTIONS

1. Preheat grill.

2. Prepare the salad dressing by combining all ingredients. Mix until smooth. Set aside.

3. Place salmon in a meat grinder or food processor. Grind or chop to ground-beef consistency. Add tamari, tapioca starch, and black pepper and grind or chop together. Form ground salmon into 4 patties, about ½ cup each. Cover and set aside in refrigerator.

4. Spray both sides of pineapple slices with canola oil and place on grill just until marked on both sides. Dice grilled pineapple and place in a medium bowl. Add remaining ingredients for salsa. Mix and set aside.

5. Grill salmon patties for 3 to 5 minutes on each side to desired doneness.

6. Place ½ cup mixed greens on each of four plates. Evenly divide the salsa and place on top of the greens. Top each salad with a salmon patty.

7. Drizzle 2 tablespoons wasabi dressing over each salad and serve.

NUTRITION INFORMATION PER SERVING

290 calories

15 g carbohydrate

11 g fat

51 mg cholesterol

20 g protein

210 mg sodium

4 g fiber

Dinner

PASTA MIAMI WITH GRILLED CHICKEN

Makes 4 servings

This Mediterranean-inspired dish is completely satisfying and easy to prepare. It also supports brain health on many fronts with whole grains, vegetables, and low-fat protein.

INGREDIENTS

Canola oil spray

1 pound Roma tomatoes
  (approximately 5 tomatoes)

2 cups whole-grain penne pasta

Four 4-ounce boneless, skinless
  chicken breasts

1 cup kale

¼ cup shallots, minced

1 tablespoon garlic, minced

2 cups vegetable stock

2 teaspoons lemon zest

½ cup feta cheese

¼ cup sliced kalamata olives

DIRECTIONS

1. Preheat oven to 400°F. Lightly spray a baking sheet with canola spray. Slice tomatoes in half and place on baking sheet sliced side up. Roast for 45 to 50 minutes or until tomatoes begin to brown and caramelize. Remove from oven, cool slightly, and cut lengthwise into thin strips.

2. Bring a large pot of water to a boil and cook pasta according to package directions. At the same time, preheat grill or broiler. Grill the chicken until it reaches an internal temperature of 165°F, approximately 4 to 5 minutes on each side.

3. Spray kale with canola oil spray and grill just until the edges begin to turn brown, a few seconds on each side.

4. Spray a sauté pan with canola oil spray. Sauté shallots and garlic until tender. Add kale and roasted tomatoes. Deglaze pan with vegetable stock and cook for an additional 2 to 3 minutes. Add pasta and cook an additional 1 to 2 minutes or until heated through.

5. Remove from heat and stir in lemon zest, feta cheese, and kalamata olives.

6. Evenly divide pasta onto 4 plates. Top each serving with one chicken breast.

NUTRITION INFORMATION PER SERVING

350 calories

30 g carbohydrate

9 g fat

91 mg cholesterol

36 g protein

531 mg sodium

2 g fiber

SESAME-CRUSTED SALMON TERIYAKI

Makes 4 servings

Sesame seeds are particularly high in folic acid, an important B vitamin necessary for brain health.

INGREDIENTS

For the Teriyaki Marinade

1 cup apple juice concentrate
½ cup low-sodium tamari sauce
¼ cup rice vinegar
¼ cup fresh lime juice
1 tablespoon garlic, minced
1 tablespoon fresh ginger, minced
1 teaspoon red pepper flakes

1 pound fresh salmon fillets, cut into 4 equal portions
1 tablespoon sesame seeds
1 tablespoon black sesame seeds
¼ teaspoon sea salt
1 tablespoon sesame oil

DIRECTIONS

1. Preheat oven to 400°F. Combine all ingredients for marinade in a medium bowl.

2. Place salmon in glass baking dish and pour marinade over salmon. Cover and marinate in the refrigerator for 10 minutes to 1 hour. Meanwhile, combine sesame seeds and salt on a plate.

3. Remove salmon from marinade and coat each piece in sesame seeds.

4. Heat sesame oil in a pan over medium-high heat. Sear salmon for 1 minute on each side, then place in oven for 5 to 10 minutes, depending on how you prefer your salmon cooked.

NUTRITION INFORMATION PER SERVING

250 calories

12 g carbohydrate

13 g fat

54 mg cholesterol

21 g protein

493 mg sodium

1 g fiber

VEGETARIAN BEAN CHILI

Makes ten 1-cup servings

Beans promote brain health because they are so high in both fiber and protein. However, they don't agree with everyone. That's why we add epazote to our chili. Epazote is an herb from Mexico that is used specifically for cooking beans and is said to have an antiflatulent effect. Epazote is also sold under the following names: wormseed, Jesuit's tea, Mexican tea, or paico. It can be purchased from specialty food stores and on the Internet.

INGREDIENTS

½ cup dried garbanzo beans
½ cup dried navy beans
½ cup dried black beans
½ cup dried adzuki beans
Pinch epazote (optional)
1 tablespoon extra virgin olive oil
1 teaspoon garlic, minced
⅔ cup red onion, diced
½ cup red bell pepper, diced
½ cup yellow bell pepper, diced
¾ teaspoon dried basil
Pinch ground cumin
1½ teaspoons chili powder
Pinch chipotle pepper powder
¼ teaspoon dried oregano

Pinch freshly ground black pepper
2½ cups canned diced tomatoes, including liquid
3 tablespoons canned tomato puree
1¾ cups tomato sauce
2 cups vegetable stock
¼ cup canned chopped green chiles
2 tablespoons fresh cilantro, chopped
1 tablespoon fresh parsley, chopped
2 teaspoons molasses
½ teaspoon sea salt

DIRECTIONS

1. Soak beans overnight. Drain water. Add fresh water. Bring to a boil and add epazote. Reduce heat and simmer for 1½ hours.

2. In a saucepan, heat olive oil over medium-high heat and sauté garlic, onion, and peppers until tender. Add dried spices and sauté briefly. Add diced tomato, tomato puree, and vegetable stock and bring to a boil. Reduce heat to low and add beans and green chiles. Simmer for 45 minutes.

3. Add cilantro, parsley, and molasses and cook for 5 minutes. Season with salt before serving.

NUTRITION INFORMATION PER SERVING

175 calories

32 g carbohydrate

2 g fat

0 mg cholesterol

9 g protein

189 mg sodium

7 g fiber

Snacks/Dessert

PEANUT BUTTER DELIGHT SPREAD

Makes ten 2-tablespoon servings

Make this ahead of time for a quick high-protein treat whenever you want something sweet. You can store this in the refrigerator for up to 1 week. It's best spread on toast or a muffin.

INGREDIENTS

> 1 cup nonfat ricotta cheese
> 2 teaspoons vanilla extract
> ½ teaspoon ground cinnamon
> 1½ tablespoons cane sugar
> ¼ cup natural peanut butter (without added salt)

DIRECTIONS

Combine all ingredients in a blender and puree until smooth. Chill in refrigerator until ready to use.

NUTRITION INFORMATION PER SERVING

65 calories
5 g carbohydrate
3 g fat
2 mg cholesterol
5 g protein
12 mg sodium
Trace fiber

WALNUT-STUFFED APPLE

Makes 6 servings

This is an elegant dessert worth serving at any family gathering. You'll also know that you are taking care of your family by treating them to something sweet and healthful at the same time. The walnuts in this recipe are particularly brain friendly: they have higher-quality antioxidants than any other nut and contain a number of potentially neuroprotective compounds, including vitamin E, folate, melatonin, and omega-3 fatty acids.

INGREDIENTS

3 Red Delicious apples

1 tablespoon pure maple syrup

1 tablespoon rolled oats

3 teaspoons unsalted butter

½ teaspoon ground cinnamon

½ teaspoon pure vanilla extract, divided

2 tablespoons brown sugar

¼ cup chopped walnuts

1 teaspoon powdered sugar

2 tablespoons heavy cream

6 sprigs fresh mint

DIRECTIONS

1. Preheat oven to 350°F.

2. Slice each apple lengthwise, remove core, and hollow out center to create a cavity for the stuffing.

3. In a small bowl, combine maple syrup, rolled oats, butter, cinnamon, ¼ teaspoon vanilla extract, brown sugar, and walnuts. Place 1½ teaspoons of filling in each apple.

4. Bake the apples in an oven-safe dish for 30 to 45 minutes until firm but tender. Let apples sit for at least 10 minutes.

5. Meanwhile combine remaining vanilla, powdered sugar, and heavy cream. Whip with whisk until soft peaks form.

6. Place one half apple on a plate and top with 1 teaspoon of cream and garnish with a sprig of mint. Repeat for each half apple.

NUTRITION INFORMATION PER SERVING

140 calories

19 g carbohydrate

7 g fat

11 mg cholesterol

2 g protein

5 mg sodium

2 g fiber

FIBER-RICH CHOCOLATE BARS

Makes 6 bars

This delicious indulgence is actually working for your brain: lots of antioxidants in the berries and the chocolate, and a significant amount of fiber and protein in the almonds.

INGREDIENTS

6 ounces dark chocolate

½ cup dried cranberries

½ cup dried blueberries

½ cup puffed quinoa or puffed rice cereal

¼ cup chopped almonds

DIRECTIONS

1. Melt chocolate using a double boiler method, stirring constantly.

2. Remove from heat and stir in cranberries, blueberries, puffed cereal, and almonds.

3. Spoon ¼-cup portions onto parchment or wax paper. Refrigerate until firm.

NUTRITION INFORMATION PER SERVING

235 calories

29 g carbohydrate

12 g fat

2 mg cholesterol

3 g protein

5 mg sodium

2 g fiber

Chapter 13

SELECT SUPPLEMENT OPTIONS

When it comes to nutrition, there is no question that whole foods have a greater positive effect than any individual supplement. Whole foods work synergistically, which means that the colors on your plate, or the ingredients in any one dish, all contain different chemical compounds that work together to create the greatest impact. For example, there is much stronger data supporting the effectiveness of antioxidants found in food than there is for pills; you are better off eating a tomato than supplementing with lycopene, because the tomato also contains vitamin C, fiber, and other important components that both your brain and your body need for optimal health. What's more, when you eat tomatoes together with other nutrient-dense foods, you are getting their benefits as well.

Blueberries offer another excellent example of how whole foods provide the greatest nutritional opportunities. The late James Joseph, PhD, was a pioneer in research on antioxidants. His research team discovered that berries, and possibly walnuts, activate the brain's natural "housekeeper" mechanism, which cleans up and recycles toxic proteins linked to age-related memory loss and other mental decline. They also identified the natural compounds called *polyphenolics* found in fruits, vegetables, and nuts, which have both an antioxidant and an anti-inflammatory effect that protects the brain. Once they identified the positive attributes of blueberries, Joseph and his team tried to determine exactly which part of the blueberry had the highest concentration of antioxidants: the skin, the fleshy fiber, or the juice. In testing each component individually, they found that no single form was as potent as the whole blueberry. So while highly concentrated forms of blueberry have been developed and can be effective antioxidants, in Dr. Joseph's words, you're better off "eating the damn blueberry."

However, there are times when you may need to use nutritional supplements in addition to following a healthy diet as outlined in chapter 6. If you know you are significantly and clinically deficient in a particular vitamin or mineral—the nutrients that the body needs to work properly—supplementing is the most efficient way to increase your intake of that particular nutrient. Discuss any symptoms you may be experiencing with your doctor—who can then order the proper testing to determine if you have any sort of vitamin or mineral deficiency.

Supplements may also be required if you have food allergies or food intolerances or are following a vegan or another restricted diet. These scenarios may prevent you from getting particular nutrients that can support brain health. For example, if you are lactose intolerant, it might be harder to get enough calcium, magnesium, or vitamin D from your diet, since you are avoiding dairy products. Last, there are some nutrients that you simply need more of than you can ever get from even the best nutritional plan. Vitamin D is a good example of this, and we'll discuss it in more detail later in the chapter.

Even if you are not experiencing symptoms or signs of illness, it's always best to talk with your doctor or nutritionist before you begin any type of supplementation program. While we know that supplements provide some benefits for brain health, it's unclear if supplements work better for those who are eating a lousy diet, or if they are giving an extra benefit or boost to those who are following a preventive health and fitness program like the one outlined in this book. What's more, some supplements can actually do more harm than good if you are combining them with medications or if you are taking them in the wrong dosages.

At Canyon Ranch we also believe that your current health status is the most important indication of what role supplements can play to prevent or delay symptoms of poor brain health. If you fall into a high-risk category for developing Alzheimer's disease, then you may need to do more than the person who is at lower risk, so supplementation may be necessary. As we discussed, the four major risk factors of Alzheimer's disease are referred to as the Four As:

- *Age*: The likelihood of developing Alzheimer's doubles every ten years after age sixty-five; after age eighty-five, the risk reaches nearly 50 percent.
- The presence of the *APOE4* gene.
- A diagnosis of *atherosclerosis,* or hardening of the arteries.
- Inflammation, most commonly seen in *arthritis,* but also seen in other systemic inflammatory disorders.

Last, keep in mind that taking supplements does not give you a free pass to revert back to bad habits; they are not an antidote to eating an entire pepperoni pizza and are not a magic pill that will keep your brain cognitively active, no matter what you've seen or heard in the media. To achieve optimal brain health, you need to consistently eat right, exercise both your brain and your body, sleep, avoid pollutants, and reduce stress. Simply put, supplements can be an important component for achieving better brain health, but they are not going to do all the hard work for you.

BEFORE YOU BUY

Unlike prescription or over-the-counter medicines, supplements exist as an underenforced niche market. There are hundreds of companies all over the world that produce supplements, and the quality among them varies greatly. What's more, their labels and product information can be intentionally confusing. On a typical visit to your local chain drugstore or even a "health store," you might find yourself looking at five different brands of vitamin D, ten dosage options, and a handful of formulations. How do you know which to choose?

Some experts recommend that you always go with the most expensive option because it's likely to have the highest-quality ingredients.

That logic might work in some instances, but not in others. At Canyon Ranch, we rely on the best outside governance available and recommend formulations that carry a USP certification that you can clearly see on the product's label. USP stands for United States Pharmacopeial, a scientific nonprofit organization that sets standards for medicines, food ingredients, and dietary supplements. Its seal of approval confirms that there has been standardization of the ingredients for that particular supplement.

You can also confirm if a particular supplement has passed some type of quality control process through independent companies that provide this service. These companies have created databases resulting in developing standards within this industry. A good example is ConsumerLab.com, and while it doesn't test all the products on the market, it does test a good number of them and rates a broad spectrum of brands and the products within those brands. It is also a great resource for the latest information and clinical studies regarding supplementation. In addition, supplements manufactured in California must meet the stringent state requirements.

When you're ready to make a purchase, look for supplements from a brand that you trust. Buy small quantities, replace them frequently, and pay attention to their expiration dates. For example, antioxidant supplements will actually oxidize over time right in the bottle, owing to exposure to oxygen. If you've got an antioxidant supplement sitting on a shelf for nine months, it's going to oxidize, no matter how dark and airtight the package. So if you buy the bottle of five hundred pills, it's going to take you six months to get through them, and most likely many will spoil before you take them.

THE BEST SUPPLEMENTS THAT SUPPORT BRAIN HEALTH

The following is a very short list of nutrients that have been clinically shown in some patients to enhance brain health and may reverse symptoms of cognitive decline. Achieving the proper levels of these nutrients is crucial for maintaining brain health. Talk with your doctor about defining specific dosages that are right for you.

Vitamin B

There are many different kinds of B vitamins: thiamine (B_1), riboflavin (B_2), niacin (B_3), folate, pantothenic acid (B_5), pyridoxine (B_6), and vitamin B^{12} (cobalamin). Some B's are especially important for the brain, and of all of them, vitamin B_{12} is probably the most significant. Vitamin B_{12} is involved in several key metabolic processes that directly affect the peripheral and central nervous system. If the brain nerve fibers and cells degenerate due to a deficiency, that may contribute to cognitive decline. Most deficiency is first manifested in the peripheral nervous system and is associated with loss of reflexes, numbness, and tingling.

We also know that a B_{12} deficiency can cause dementia, and with proper supplementation, you can reverse this condition. Folate, or folic acid, is also necessary to support brain health. The Baltimore Longitudinal Study of Aging found that people taking four hundred micrograms of folic acid had half the Alzheimer's rates compared with those who didn't take the supplement. Another 2010 study, published in the journal *Psychopharmacology,* reported that a team of British neuroscientists found a clear link between B vitamins and improving mood and cognition. In their study, men taking high-dose B-complex vitamins showed improved performance in cognitive tasks, were less mentally tired, and showed improved vigor.

A vitamin B_{12} deficiency can easily occur if you are following a vegan diet, because this nutrient is found naturally only in animal products such as meats, eggs, and poultry. People who follow a more balanced diet might still be deficient in B_{12} if they have a problem with its absorption, a condition known as *pernicious anemia.*

Thiamine is another B vitamin that's critical for the brain. Most grain products are fortified with this vitamin, but if you're cutting down on grains, you may need more thiamine. You can get B vitamins either through a multivitamin, a B-complex vitamin, or a single-nutrient supplement. When you buy a B-complex vitamin, you're typically getting all of the B's together.

Vitamin D

This essential nutrient is actually a hormone that is naturally produced in the skin. There are more than a dozen distinct types of vitamin D produced through exposure to sunlight. Some of them last for just seconds, and then are chemically converted to other forms of vitamin D that the body can use. In addition to its well-known function in calcium and bone development, vitamin D is known to be beneficial for brain health: it both protects the brain and reduces inflammation. Vitamin D has been shown to correlate with a decreased level of amyloid plaques in the brain, the same ones known to be present in Alzheimer's disease. It is also thought to combat depression and improve cognitive function. A 2012 study conducted by the University of Manchester proposed that an adequate level of vitamin D helps maintain brain health and cognitive function. Researchers found that individuals with high levels of vitamin D outperformed those with low levels in areas including memory and information processing. Another 2012 study, presented at the Endocrine Society's 94th Annual Meeting & Expo, found that women with moderate-to-severe depression had substantial improvement in their symptoms after they received treatment for vitamin D deficiency.

Vitamin D is found in fatty fish such as salmon, tuna, and sardines; fortified milk and dairy products; fortified juice; fortified cereals; and eggs. However, these food sources do not provide sufficient quantities of vitamin D to meet your daily needs. A typical dose is a thousand international units (IU) a day. However, you'd have to drink ten glasses of milk each day to get that much.

A better source of D is actually the sun, but this is effective only if you live in a warm climate where the sun is bright. If you live north of the 37th parallel, which runs horizontally from Los Angeles to Atlanta, your skin can't make vitamin D from the sun between September and May unless you live at an altitude over five thousand feet. Sun exposure has other complications, specifically increasing your risk of skin cancer or sun damage. The sunscreen that protects our skin also prevents vitamin D production.

We do recommend that whenever possible, and when you are in the right climate zone, you expose your skin to the sun for twenty minutes a day, applying sunblock to your face, chest, arms, and hands. These are the areas of the body that have typically received more than enough sun exposure over time, and the most likely places where skin cancers can develop. However, you can skip the sunscreen on your back, legs, and feet for the first twenty minutes, and then apply it if you are spending the day in the sun.

Because of these issues, most doctors and nutritionists agree that the best way to ensure the right amount of vitamin D is actually through supplementation. There are two types of vitamin D supplements, D_2 and D_3. D_2 is the plant form; D_3 is the animal form. Each is effective (although D_2 does not raise blood serum levels as quickly), but the dosages are different—another reason why it's important to talk with your health care provider before you start shopping for vitamins.

Fish Oil

Omega-3s are critical for brain health and, as you learned in chapter 6, are highly concentrated in cold-water fatty fish and in some nuts and seeds. However, if you are insulin resistant or diabetic, you will need to obtain the correct amounts of omega-3s from fish oil supplements, because the process of transforming ALA into EPA can be blocked in the presence of high insulin levels. The two types of omega-3 oils found in fish are EPA (eicosapentaenoic acid) and DHA (docosahexaenoic acid). These fats actually originate from ocean algae and are concentrated in the food chain as fish eat the algae and are then eaten by bigger fish.

Look for fish oil supplements that are in a liquid or a soft gel form and are derived from harvested fish caught in deep waters far removed from major shipping lanes. The best sources are also "molecularly distilled" fish oils that have been tested for PCBs, heavy metals, and particularly mercury. There are dozens of different types of fish oil, let alone brands and formulations. The third-party resource Canyon Ranch uses for choosing fish oil supplements is the International Fish Oil Standards Program (IFOS). The IFOS criteria for determining fish oil quality were established by the World Health Organization (WHO) and the Council for Responsible Nutrition (CRN). Look for the IFOS seal of approval when you are shopping for this supplement.

On the supplement label, look for the letters EPA and DHA, which refer to the milligrams of omega-3s in each serving. The total amounts of both EPA and DHA should be at least a thousand milligrams.

Healthy Omega-6 Choices

Although omega-6 fats sometimes worsen inflammation, one omega-6 fatty acid can be transformed into anti-inflammatory eicosanoids. Gamma-linolenic acid (GLA), an intermediate fatty acid in the conversion of linoleic acid to arachidonic acid, is transformed first into dihomo-gamma-linolenic acid (DGLA) and then into anti-inflammatory eicosanoids. It can also be obtained from evening primrose oil, borage, and black currant oil.

Antioxidants

In chapter 6 we discussed the link between dietary antioxidants and reducing the risk of Alzheimer's disease. Researchers believe that these nutrients work synergistically with one another to offer the greatest protection for your brain, and therefore we recommend taking an antioxidant formulation that contains many compounds, instead of supplementing only one type at a time. In a study released from Oregon Health & Science University, researchers found that taking an antioxidant formula containing vitamins B, C, D, and E was associated with better cognitive function and larger brain volume. They found that even though vitamin E (especially in the form *gamma-tocopherol*) is thought to improve cognitive function and may delay the onset of Alzheimer's disease, supplementation of this nutrient by itself didn't yield a positive outcome. The same was true for vitamin C, which is thought to play an important role in the synthesis of norepinephrine, a neurotransmitter critical to brain function and mood regulation. However, when vitamin C was combined with vitamin E, the results were positive.

Do You Overproduce Nuclear Factor-Kappa B (NF-kB)?

Some individuals are genetically prone to increased inflammation and may have increased levels of the protein nuclear factor-kappa B (NF-kB). This protein increases the activity of genes that raise inflammation. For example, NF-kB is elevated in those with rheumatoid arthritis. If you have been diagnosed with this or any other inflammatory disease, supplementing with alpha-lipoic acid, vitamin C, and flavonoids has been shown to help inhibit NF-kB activity. Talk to your doctor about these options.

Resveratrol

Resveratrol is a specific type of antioxidant found in the skins of dark berries and grapes. It's thought to be one of the beneficial nutrients in red wine. Resveratrol is in a class of polyphenols called *sirtuin,* which is a gene activator. It has been found to help repair genes and make them more resistant to damage, thereby increasing neuroplasticity by decreasing cellular death.

However, you'd have to drink a lot of red wine to increase your intake of resveratrol, and with that comes another trade-off. Any type of alcoholic beverage is considered to be a *neurotoxin*: it kills brain cells. While one glass of wine daily may be protective, having more than two glasses a day may actually make things worse. If you want the benefits of resveratrol without the negative side effects of alcohol, supplementation might be your best bet.

Probiotics

Probiotics are a class of nutritional supplement known to balance immune function and decrease inflammation, which again is one of the risk factors for Alzheimer's disease. These healthy bacteria maintain an environment in the intestinal tract and are also beneficial in reducing inflammation throughout the brain and the body.

Probiotics are most effective when they are combined with a high-fiber diet or a fiber supplement. The fiber acts as the fertilizer that makes the probiotics grow. And because probiotics interact with the digestive system, each strain performs differently depending on your gut's unique environment. This means that one type of probiotic doesn't work the same for everybody.

In order to find the supplement that will work best for you, choose a broad-spectrum, high-potency probiotic combined with fiber. *Broad spectrum* means that it contains more than one strain of probiotics. You might also want to try different formulations in order to find the one that works best for you.

Turmeric

The same spice that gives curries their bright yellow color and spicy flavor also combats inflammation because it is an inhibitor of an enzyme called *COX* 2. Turmeric is currently being studied by the National Institutes of Health (NIH) for a possible role in lowering the risk of Alzheimer's disease. What's more, it is known to be an effective blocker of TNF alpha, a naturally occurring chemical that has been implicated in a variety of human diseases, including Alzheimer's disease and rheumatoid arthritis. Turmeric is also thought to stimulate the production of acetylcholine and break up amyloid plaques.

However, you need more than a dusting on your foods to get these important health benefits, and this is why a turmeric supplement may be as good as, or even better than, liberally using the spice in your cooking.

Start Low and Go Slow

When it comes to vitamins and minerals, more is not always better. At Canyon Ranch, our philosophy for nutrient supplementation is as follows: "Start low and go slow." Ask your doctor to suggest the smallest effective dosage of a particular supplement and see if there is a way that you can start low and build up, and then schedule an appointment to come back a few weeks later to determine its effectiveness. See if you notice a shift in your thinking or mood so you can tell if the supplement will be beneficial over the short term or the long term. If you are compensating for a vitamin deficiency, you might have to take specific supplements for a long time before your levels return to a normal range.

You may also want to consider taking one type of supplement at a time: don't overload your system by taking handfuls of vitamins together. If you find that you are deficient in lots of vitamins, consider taking a multivitamin that covers many of the nutrients outlined in the chapter, as well as others that promote overall health. Then go back to chapter 6 to see how you can add more nutrients into your eating plan to have the greatest impact on your brain health.

Chapter 14

———

A PERFECT DAY OF
BRAIN HEALTH

By now you should have a complete understanding of everything you need to do to support and enhance your brain's health. Medicine, diet, exercise, spirituality, and behavioral modification all play equal roles. The last step is integrating them into one seamless program: a perfect day of brain health.

You don't need to give up your job and your life in order to devote your attention to your brain. Taking care of yourself can be easily worked into your day, and by following these guidelines you will be incorporating all of the information, tips, and tricks that you've just read about. And while we know you'll get the most benefits by following this strictly, we understand that not everyone can do this perfectly every day. Strive for most days at first, but once you start, you'll quickly see how much better you'll feel and think, and before long, you will have created that three-step habit loop of cue-routine-reward. Once you begin the program, you'll want to live like this every day. Ultimately, that's what Canyon Ranch is all about. While we like our visitors to come and stay with us, we're more impressed when they take what they've learned home and incorporate it into their daily lives.

A perfect day at Canyon Ranch begins bright and early, but we're not going to put you on the clock just yet. The following are simply good suggestions so you can organize a day of optimal living in terms of your brain health. By the time you're ready to go to work, you've done the majority of your daily health care. The practices that matter most have been done for the day, and the rest of the day is about having control. By the end of the day, you need to make sure you've incorporated the Canyon Ranch philosophy, which, again, is based on four spheres of well-being:

- The Physical: Am I taking care of my body?
- The Mental: Am I actively engaged in learning?
- The Emotional: Am I working toward balance?
- The Spiritual: Am I connected to something outside myself?

BEFORE-BREAKFAST ACTIVITY

✓ Start your day with an energizing meditation from chapter 8, taking between five and twenty minutes. Allow yourself a moment, even before your feet hit the floor, to remember that there's something bigger and broader in life.

✓ Exercise for brain health; see chapter 7 and follow the daily routine.

BREAKFAST

✓ Start your eating day with a high-protein breakfast and a handful of antioxidant-rich berries, such as blueberries. When you have a high-protein breakfast, you feel more satisfied and are less likely to snack before lunch. Eggs are a terrific choice because the whites are a complete protein and the yolks are an excellent source of omega-3s and vitamin D. Protein shakes and Greek yogurt are also excellent choices, as well as the recipes in chapter 12. This kind of breakfast is also addressing inflammation and detoxification.

✓ Don't forget the coffee, if you can tolerate it. Caffeine has been shown to inhibit plaque formation in the brain.

✓ Brush your teeth and floss to make sure you don't develop infections of the gum like periodontitis that can travel to the brain.

✓ Detoxify your body: move your bowels and drink plenty of water now and throughout the day.

Midmorning Activity

✓ Do twenty minutes of brain-gym exercises to keep your mind active and learning new things. Or take a quick break with a challenging piece of fiction or a magazine article that requires a close read.

Lunch

✓ Small, healthy meals throughout the day maintain good blood-sugar levels and supply your brain glucose in a smooth and even way.

✓ Think about the Japanese saying *Hara hachi bu*, which means "Eat till you're 80 percent full." Eighty percent full is going to be different for each of us, but it is important to implement; when you overeat beyond what your body can process, digest, assimilate, and distribute evenly, you overwhelm the system, causing oxidative stress.

Midafternoon Activity

✓ Perform a mindfulness practice to refocus your attention. A second twenty-minute meditation segment can help you become more productive, particularly in the late afternoon.

Dinner

✓ As you focus on the last meal of the day, make sure it includes lots of healthy antioxidant-rich foods. Treat yourself to one of the special recipes listed in chapter 12, and use your time cooking as an opportunity to be creative or to try something new.

Evening Activity

✓ Turn off the electronics and begin to unwind. It wasn't so long ago that we all survived in a world without smartphones and instant Internet access. Use your time in the evening to see friends or get out and socialize.

✓ Try one of the many stress-relieving activities listed in chapter 3 before you turn in for the night. Change them frequently so you can find just the right one for you.

Bedtime

✓ Brush your teeth a second time.

✓ Do a breathing practice that increases oxygenation and improves overall brain health.

✓ Get at least seven hours of uninterrupted sleep to rest and reset your brain.

THE PRACTICE IS MORE IMPORTANT THAN PERFECTION

Our goal for you is simple: to put you on the path toward better brain health, but not to insist on perfection. There will be plenty of days when you aren't able to eat perfectly or have the perfect workout. But every minute of every day counts toward moving your health forward, because something is always more than nothing.

All the elements of this program combine into a practice of healthy living that's meant to be additive to your life. Honor that place, and remember all the people who are following the same path you are. Share with your friends and family what you've learned, so that you can work together toward a healthier lifestyle.

Last, allow yourself to know that success is in you. Perfection will take you away from this knowledge, but the experience of following the program to the best of your ability will bring you closer. Every day, you want to positively increase the things that are good for your body as well as the things that are going to slow down your brain's aging. And then as you move forward, you want to keep those good habits going, because good habits beget more good habits. Before you know it, you will have achieved a perfect day.

Acknowledgments

Canyon Ranch is an integrative experience because our specialists work together every day to bring the best of health care to our guests. This effort has continued in creating this book. I am grateful to Mark Liponis, MD; Param Dedhia, MD; Stephen Brewer, MD; Cindy Geyer, MD; Tereza Hubkova, MD; Karen Koffler, MD; Diane Downing, MD; and Allan J. Hamilton, MD, FACS, for generously providing their medical expertise and insights to help create this book. Jeff Rossman, PhD; Ann Pardo MA, LPC, ACS, NCGC; Julie Haber; and Karen McIntyre, MSW, were integral in the creation of the stress management, spirituality, and meditation chapters; exercise physiologists Mike Siemens, MS; and Rich Butler, MS, CSCS, supplied not only their insights but the latest scientific findings to create an exercise chapter that truly promotes brain health. Nutritionists Lisa Powell, MS, RD; Christine Sardo, PhD, MPH, RD; and Chef Scott Uehlein were instrumental in providing accurate information on nutrition and wonderful recipes that capture all we do at Canyon Ranch. Last, acupuncturist Kelly Ann Clady-Giramma, LAc, Dipl OM; and Gary Schwartz, PhD, shared their expertise regarding alternative therapies.

I could not have written this book without the help of my staff and the professional staff at Canyon Ranch, Tucson: thanks to Patricia Maxwell, Carrie Kennedy, and Ramona Durrer for making the creation of this book a smooth and organized process. Jude McCarthy, Tucson general manager Kyle Treat, and Lenox general manager Reggie Cooper made navigating the various properties effortless. Thanks to

Christie Hefner and Marjorie Martin for their coordination, guidance, and input. Mel and Enid Zuckerman, as well as Jerry Cohen, provided the inspiration for the book.

I had a fantastic experience with my publishing team at Atria Books, including my editor Sarah Durand and publisher Judith Curr. Illustrator Karen Morgenbesser crafted drawings that make the intricacies of the brain easy to understand. Pam Liflander was our literary guide and served as the glue that brought all the content together, while making the process fun.

And last but certainly not least, huge thanks to my family, who supported me in this endeavor and realized that as I aged, this book was as much for me as for everyone else.

Resources and Suggested Reading

Boyce, Barry, ed., with the editors of the *Shambhala Sun*. *The Mindfulness Revolution: Leading Psychologists, Scientists, Artists, and Meditation Teachers on the Power of Mindfulness in Daily Life*. Boston: Shambhala Publications, Inc., 2011.

Brewer, Stephen C., and Peggy Holt Wagner. *The Everest Principle: How to Achieve the Summit of Your Life*. Carlsbad, Calif.: Hay House, 2010.

Colborn, Theo, Dianne Dumanoski, and John Peterson Myers. *Our Stolen Future: Are We Threatening Our Fertility, Intelligence, and Survival? A Scientific Detective Story*. New York: Dutton, 1996.

Katie, Byron, and Stephen Mitchell. *Loving What Is: Four Questions That Can Change Your Life*. New York: Harmony Books, 2002.

Morrison, Jeffrey A. *Cleanse Your Body, Clear Your Mind: Eliminate Environmental Toxins to Lose Weight, Increase Energy, and Reverse Illness in 30 Days or Less*. New York: Hudson Street Press, 2011.

Ratey, John J. *A User's Guide to the Brain: Perception, Attention, and the Four Theaters of the Brain*. New York: Vintage Books, 2002.

Rossman, Jeffrey. *The Mind-Body Mood Solution: The Breakthrough Drug-Free Program for Lasting Relief from Depression*. New York: Rodale, 2011.

Schwartz, Gary E., with William L. Simon. *The Energy Healing Experiments: Science Reveals Our Natural Power to Heal*. New York: Atria Books, 2008.

Snowdon, David. *Aging with Grace: What the Nun Study Teaches Us about Leading Longer, Healthier, and More Meaningful Lives*. New York: Bantam Books, 2001.

References

Chapter 1

Gougoux, Frédéric, Robert J. Zatorre, Maryse Lassonde, Patrice Voss, and Franco Lepore. "A Functional Neuroimaging Study of Sound Localization: Visual Cortex Activity Predicts Performance in Early-Blind Individuals." *PLOS Biology* 3, no. 2 (2005): E27.

Chapter 2

Christensen, Kaare, MD; Mikael Thinggaard, MSc; Anna Oksuzyan, MD; Troels Steenstrup, PhD; Karen Andersen-Ranberg, MD; Bernard Jeune, MD; Matt McGue, PhD; and James W. Vaupel PhD. "Physical and Cognitive Functioning of People Older Than 90 years: A Comparison of Two Danish Cohorts Born 10 Years Apart." *The Lancet,* July 11, 2013. DOI: 10.1016/S0140-6736(13)60777-1.

Epperson, C. Neill, Zenab Amin, Kosha Ruparel, Ruben Gur, and James Loughead. "Interactive Effects of Estrogen and Serotonin on Brain Activation During Working Memory and Affective Processing in Menopausal Women." *Psychoneuroendocrinology* 37, no. 3 (March 2012): 372–82.

Gräff, J., D. Kim, M. M. Dobbin, and L. H. Tsai. "Epigenetic Regulation of Gene Expression in Physiological and Pathological Brain Processes." *Physiological Reviews* 91, no. 2 (April 2011): 603–49.

Holland, J., S. Bandelow, and E. Hogervorst. "Testosterone Levels and Cognition in Elderly Men: A Review." *Maturitas* 69, no. 4 (August 2011): 322–37.

Lu, T., Y. Pan, S. Y. Kao, C. Li, I. Kohane, J. Chan, and B. A. Yankner. "Gene Regulation and DNA Damage in the Ageing Human Brain." *Nature* 429, no. 6994 (June 24, 2004): 883–91.

Matthews, Fiona E., PhD; Antony Arthur, PhD; Linda E. Barnes, RGN; John Bond, BA; Carol Jagger, PhD; Louise Robinson, MD; and Carol Brayne, MD. "A Two-Decade Comparison of Prevalence of Dementia in Individuals Aged 65 Years and Older from Three Geographical Areas of England: Results of the Cognitive Function and Ageing Study I and II." *The Lancet,* July 17, 2013. DOI: 10.1016/S0140-6736(13)61570-6.

McCullough, Louise D., and Patricia D. Hurn. "Estrogen and Ischemic Neuroprotection: An Integrated View." *Trends in Endocrinology & Metabolism* 14, no. 5 (July 2003): 228–35.

Naj, Adam C., et al. "Common Variants at MS4A4/MS4A6E, CD2AP, CD33 and EPHA1 Are Associated with Late-Onset Alzheimer's Disease." *Nature Genetics* 43, no. 5 (May 2011): 436–41, doi: 10.1038/ng.801.

Chapter 3

Heffernan, Tom, and Terence O'Neill. "A Comparison of Social (Weekend) Smokers, Regular (Daily) Smokers and a Never-Smoked Group upon Everyday Prospective Memory." *The Open Addiction Journal* 4, no. 1 (2011): 72–75, doi: 10.2174/1874941001104010072.

Hou, Wen-Hsuan, MD, MSc; Pai-Tsung Chiang, MD, MPH; Tun-Yen Hsu, MD; Su-Ying Chiu, BA; and Yung-Chieh Yen, MD, MSc, PhD. "Treatment Effects of Massage Therapy in Depressed People: A Meta-Analysis." *Journal of Clinical Psychiatry* 71, no. 7 (2010): 894–901, doi: 10.4088/JCP.09r05009blu.

Sheline, Yvette I., Mokhtar H. Gado, and Helena C. Kraemer. "Untreated Depression and Hippocampal Volume Loss." *American Journal of Psychiatry* 160 (2003): 1516–18, doi: 10.1176/appi.ajp.160.8.1516.

Chapter 4

Ancelin, M. L., et al. "Long-Term Post-Operative Cognitive Decline in the Elderly: The Effects of Anesthesia Type, Apolipoprotein E Genotype, and Clinical Antecedents," supplement, *Journal of Alzheimer's Disease* 22, no. S3 (2010): 105–13, doi: 10.3233/JAD-2010-100807.

Keller, J. N., et al. "Evidence of Increased Oxidative Damage in Subjects with Mild Cognitive Impairment." *Neurology* 64, no. 7 (April 12, 2005): 1152–56.

Onstot, Jon D., Randall E. Ayling, and John S. Stanley. "Characterization of HRGC/MS Unidentified Peaks from the Analysis of Human Adipose Tissue: Volume 1, Technical Approach." Washington, D.C.: U.S. Environmental Protection Agency Office of Pesticides and Toxic Substances, 1987.

Rasmussen, L. S. "Postoperative Cognitive Dysfunction: Incidence and Prevention." *Best Practice & Research Clinical Anaesthesiology* 20, no. 2 (June 2006): 315–30.

Shubert, Jack, E. Joan Riley, and Sylvanus A. Tyler. "Combined Effects in Toxicology—A Rapid Systematic Testing Procedure: Cadmium, Mercury, and Lead." *Journal of Toxicology and Environmental Health* 4, no. 5–6 (1978): 763–76, doi: 10.1080/15287397809529698.

Straus, D. C. "Molds, Mycotoxins, and Sick Building Syndrome." *Toxicology and Industrial Health* 25, no. 9–10 (October/November 2009): 617–35, doi: 10.1177/0748233709348287.

Wang, Anthony, Sadie Costello, Myles Cockburn, Xinbo Zhang, Jeff Bronstein, and Beate Ritz. "Parkinson's Disease Risk from Ambient Exposure to Pesticides." *European Journal of Epidemiology* 26, no. 7 (July 1, 2011): 547–55.

Weiss, Bernard. "Endocrine Disruptors as a Threat to Neurological Function." *Journal of the Neurological Sciences* 305, no. 1–2 (June 15, 2011): 11–21.

Weuve, Jennifer, MPH, ScD; Robin C. Puett, MPH, PhD; Joel Schwartz, PhD; Jeff D. Yanosky, MS, ScD; Francine Laden, MS, ScD; and Francine Grodstein, ScD. "Exposure to Particulate Air Pollution and Cognitive Decline in Older Women." *Archives of Internal Medicine* 172, no. 3 (February 13, 2012): 219–27, doi:10.1001/archinternmed.2011.683.

Chapter 5

Attele, Anoja S., DDS; Jing-Tian Xie, MD; and Chun-Su Yuan, MD, PhD. "Treatment of Insomnia: An Alternative Approach." *Alternative Medicine Review* 5, no. 3 (2000): 249–59.

Décary, Anne, PhD; Isabelle Rouleau, PhD; and Jacques Montplaisir, MD, FRCPc, PhD. "Cognitive Deficits Associated with Sleep Apnea Syndrome: A Proposed Neuropsychological Test Battery." *Sleep* 23, no. 3 (2000): 369–81.

Joo, Eun Yeon, et al. "Reduced Brain Gray Matter Concentration in Patients with Obstructive Sleep Apnea Syndrome." *Sleep* 33, no. 2 (February 2010): 235–41.

Karni, A., D. Tanne, B. S. Rubenstein, J. J. Askenasy, and D. Sagi. "Dependence on REM Sleep of Overnight Improvement of a Perceptual Skill." *Science* 265, no. 5172 (July 29, 1994): 679–82, doi: 10.1126/science.8036518.

Morin, Charles M., PhD; Cheryl Colecchi, PhD; Jackie Stone, PhD; Rakesh Sood, MD; and Douglas Brink, PharmD. "Behavioral and Pharmacological Therapies for Late-Life Insomnia." *Journal of the American Medical Association* 28, no. 11 (March 17, 1999): 991–9, doi:10.1001/jama.281.11.991.

Walker, Matthew P. "Cognitive Consequences of Sleep and Sleep Loss," supplement, *Sleep Medicine* 9, no. S1 (2008): S29–34.

Yaffe, Kristine, MD, et al. "Sleep-Disordered Breathing, Hypoxia, and Risk of Mild Cognitive Impairment and Dementia in Older Women." *Journal of the American Medical Association* 306, no. 6 (August 10, 2011): 613–19, doi:10.1001/jama.2011.1115.

Chapter 6

Crichton, G. E., M. F. Elias, G. A. Dore, M. A. Robbins. "Relation Between Dairy Food Intake and Cognitive Function: The Maine-Syracuse Longitudinal Study." *International Dairy Journal* 22, no. 1 (January 2012): 15–23.

Fischera, Karina, Paolo C. Colombania, Wolfgang Langhansb, and Caspar Wenka. "Carbohydrate to Protein Ratio in Food and Cognitive Performance in the Morning." *Physiology & Behavior* 75, no. 3 (March 2002): 411–23.

Gardener, Hannah, ScD; Nikolaos Scarmeas, MD, MS; Yian Gu, PhD; Bernadette Boden-Albala, MPH, DrPh; Mitchell S. V. Elkind, MD, MS; Ralph L. Sacco, MD, MS; Charles DeCarli, MD; and Clinton B. Wright, MD, MS. "Mediterranean Diet and White Matter Hyperintensity Volume in the Northern Manhattan Study." *Archives of Neurology* 69, no. 2 (2012): 251–56, doi:10.1001/archneurol.2011.548.

Johnson, Guy H., and Kevin Fritsche. "Effect of Dietary Linoleic Acid on Markers of Inflammation in Healthy Persons: A Systematic Review of Randomized Controlled Trials." *Journal of the Academy of Nutrition and Dietetics* 112, no. 7 (July 2012): 1029–41.

Letenneur, L., C. Proust-Lima, A. Le Gouge, J. F. Dartigues, and P. Barberger-Gateau. "Flavonoid Intake and Cognitive Decline over a 10-Year Period." *American Journal of Epidemiology* 165, no. 12 (June 15, 2007): 1364–71.

Morris, M. "Associations of Vegetable and Fruit Consumption with Age-Related Cognitive Change." *Neurology* 67 (October 24, 2006): 1370–76.

Mozaffarian, Dariush, Tao Hao, Eric B. Rimm, Walter C. Willett, and Frank B. Hu. "Changes in Diet and Lifestyle and Long-Term Weight Gain in Women and Men." *New England Journal of Medicine* 364, no. 25 (2011): 2392–2404, doi: 10.1056/NEJMoa1014296.

Polidori, M. Cristina, Domenico Praticó, Francesca Mangialasche, Elena Mariani, Olivier Aust, Timur Anlasik, Ni Mang, et al. "High Fruit and Vegetable Intake Is Positively Correlated with Antioxidant Status and Cognitive Performance in Healthy Subjects." *Journal of Alzheimer's Disease* 17, no. 4 (August 2009): 921–27.

Poly, Coreyann, Joseph M. Massaro, Sudha Seshadri, Philip A. Wolf, Eunyoung Cho, Elizabeth Krall, Paul F. Jacques, and Rhoda Au. "The Relation of Dietary Choline to Cognitive Performance and White-Matter Hyperintensity in the Framingham Offspring Cohort." *American Journal of Clinical Nutrition* 94, no. 6 (2011): 1584–91.

Raz, Naftali, Karen M. Rodrigue, Kristen M. Kennedy, and James D. Acker. "Vascular Health and Longitudinal Changes in Brain and Cognition in Middle-Aged and Older Adults." *Neuropsychology* 21, no. 2 (2007): 149–57.

Smith, A., C. Bazzoni, J. Beale, J. Elliott-Smith, and M. Tiley. "High Fibre Breakfast Cereals Reduce Fatigue." *Appetite* 37, 3 (December 2001): 249–50.

Stancliffe, R. A., T. Thorpe, and M. B. Zemel. "Dairy Attenuates Oxidative and Inflammatory Stress in Metabolic Syndrome." *American Journal of Clinical Nutrition* 94, no. 2 (August 2011): 422–30.

Chapter 7

Buchman, A. S., P. A. Boyle, L. Yu, R. C. Shah, R. S. Wilson, and D. A. Bennett. "Total Daily Physical Activity and the Risk of AD and Cognitive Decline in Older Adults." *Neurology* 78 (April 24, 2012): 1323–29.

Cassilhas, Ricardo C., Hanna Karen M. Antunes, Sérgio Tufik, and Marco Túlio De Mello. "Mood, Anxiety, and Serum IGF-1 in Elderly Men Given 24 Weeks of High Resistance Exercise." *Perceptual and Motor Skills* 110, no. 1 (February 2010): 265–76.

Erickson, Kirk, Michelle Voss, Ruchika Prakash, Chandramilika Basak, Amanda Szabo, Laura Chaddock, Siobhan White, et al. "Reply to Coen et al.: Exercise, Hippocampal Volume, and Memory." *Proceedings of the National Academy of Sciences of the United States of America* 108, no. 18 (May 3, 2011): E90.

Geda, Y. E., R. O. Roberts, D. S. Knopman, T. J. H. Christianson, V. S. Pankratz, R. J. Ivnik, B. F. Boeve, et al. "Physical Exercise, Aging, and Mild Cognitive Impairment: A Population-Based Study." *Archives of Neurology* 67, no. 1 (2010): 80–86.

Hillman, Charles H., Robert W. Motl, Matthew B. Pontifex, Danielle Posthuma, Janine H. Stubbe, Dorret I. Boomsma, and Eco J. C. De Geus. "Physical Activity and Cognitive Function in a Cross-Section of Younger and Older Community-Dwelling Individuals." *Health Psychology* 25, no. 6 (2006): 678–87.

Chapter 8

Hölzel, Britta K., James Carmody, Mark Vangel, Christina Congleton, Sita M. Yerramsetti, Tim Gard, and Sara W. Lazar. "Mindfulness Practice Leads to Increases in Regional Brain Gray Matter Density." *Psychiatry Research: Neuroimaging* 191, no. 1 (January 30, 2011): 36–43, doi: 10.1016/j.pscychresns.2010.08.006.

Jha, Amishi P., Elizabeth A. Stanley, Anastasia Kiyonaga, Ling Wong, and Lois Gelfand. "Examining the Protective Effects of Mindfulness Training on Working Memory Capacity and Affective Experience." *Emotion* 10, no. 1 (February 2010): 54–64.

Luders, Eileen, Arthur W. Toga, Natasha Lepore, and Christian Gaser. "The Underlying Anatomical Correlates of Long-Term Meditation: Larger Hippocampal and Frontal Volumes of Gray Matter." *NeuroImage* 45, no. 3 (2009): 672–78.

Lutz, Antoine, Julie Brefczynski-Lewis, Tom Johnstone, and Richard J. Davidson. "Regulation of the Neural Circuitry of Emotion by Compassion Meditation: Effects of Meditative Expertise." *PLOS ONE* 3, no. 3 (2008): E1897, doi:10.1371/journal.pone.0001897.

Lutz, Antoine, Lawrence L. Greischar, Nancy B. Rawlings, Matthieu Ricard, and Richard J. Davidson. "Long-Term Meditators Self-Induce High-Amplitude Gamma Synchrony During Mental Practice." *Proceedings of the National Academy of Sciences of the United States of America* 101, no. 46 (2004): 16369–73.

Zeidan, Fadel, Nakia S. Gordon, Junaid Merchant, and Paula Goolkasian. "The Effects of Brief Mindfulness Meditation Training on Experimentally Induced Pain." *The Journal of Pain* 11, no. 3 (March 2010): 199–209.

Chapter 9

Melamed, S., A. Shirom, S. Toker, S. Berliner, and I. Shapira. "Association of Fear of Terror with Low-Grade Inflammation Among Apparently Healthy Employed Adults." *Psychosomatic Medicine* 66, no. 4 (July–August 2004): 484–91.

Schmidt, R., H. Schmidt, J. D. Curb, K. Masaki, L. R. White, and L. J. Launer. "Early Inflammation and Dementia: A 25-Year Follow-Up of the Honolulu-Asia Aging Study." *Annals of Neurology* 52, no. 2 (August 2002): 168–174. doi: 10.1002/ana.10265.

Chapter 10

Parkinson, Iona, and Carole Milligan. "The Effects of Qigong Exercise Classes on People with Dementia." *Journal of Dementia Care* 19, no. 1 (January/February 2011): 33–36.

Russek, Linda G., and Gary E. Schwartz. "Interpersonal Heart-Brain Registration and the Perception of Parental Love: A 42-Year Follow-Up of the Harvard Mastery of Stress Study." *Subtle Energies & Energy Medicine* 5, no. 3 (1994): 195–208.

Wang, Chenchen, MD, MSc; Jean Paul Collet, MD, PhD; Joseph Lau, MD. "The Effect of Tai Chi on Health Outcomes in Patients with Chronic Conditions: A Systematic Review." *Archives of Internal Medicine* 164 (2004): 493.

Chapter 11

Carlson, M., J. Saczynski, G. Rebok, T. Seeman, T. Glass, S. McGill, J. Tielsch, K. Frick, J. Hill, and L. Fried. "Exploring the Effects of an 'Everyday' Activity Program on Executive Function and Memory in Older Adults: Experience Corps." *Gerontologist* 48, no. 6 (2008): 793–801.

Chertkow, Howard, MD; Victor Whitehead, MA; Natalie Phillips, PhD; Christina Wolfson, PhD; Julie Atherton, PhD; and Howard Bergman, MD. "Multilingualism (but Not Always Bilingualism) Delays the Onset of Alzheimer Disease: Evidence-from a Bilingual Community." *Alzheimer Disease & Associated Disorders* 24, no. 2 (April/June 2010): 118–25.

Dworak, Markus, Thomas Schierl, Thomas Bruns, and Heiko Klaus Strüder. "Impact of Singular Excessive Computer Game and Television Exposure on Sleep Patterns and Memory Performance of School-Aged Children." *Pediatrics* 120, no. 5 (November 1, 2007): 978–85, doi:10.1542/peds.2007-0476.

Edwards, J., P. Delahunt, and H. Mahncke. "Cognitive Speed of Processing Training Delays Driving Cessation." *Journal of Gerontology: Series A, Biological Sciences Medical Sciences* 64, no. 12 (2009): 1262–67.

Katzman, R., R. Terry, R. DeTeresa, T. Brown, P. Davies, P. Fuld, X. Renbing, and A. Peck. "Clinical, Pathological, and Neurochemical Changes in Dementia: A Subgroup with Preserved Mental Status and Numerous Neocortical Plaques." *Annals of Neurology* 23, no. 2 (1998): 138–44.

Chapter 13

Kennedy, D. O., R. Veasey, A. Watson, F. Dodd, E. Jones, S. Maggini, and C. F. Haskell. "Effects of High-Dose B Vitamin Complex with Vitamin C and Minerals on Subjective Mood and Performance in Healthy Males." *Psychopharmacology* 211, no. 1 (July 2010): 55–68.

Soni, Maya, Katarina Kos, Iain A. Lang, Kerry Jones, David Melzer, and David J. Llewellyn. "Vitamin D and Cognitive Function," supplement, *Scandinavian Journal of Clinical & Laboratory Investigation* 72, no. S243 (April 2012): 79–82.

Yu, J., M. Gattoni-Celli, H. Zhu, N. R. Bhat, K. Sambamurti, S. Gattoni-Cell, and M. S. Kindy. "Vitamin D_3-Enriched Diet Correlates with a Decrease of Amyloid Plaques in the Brain of AβPP Transgenic Mice." *Journal of Alzheimer's Disease* 25, no. 2 (2011): 295–307.

Index

Toxins (*cont.*)
dietary, 64, 74–75
in the home, 71–72
from medications and medical
procedures, 73–74
testing for, 213, 214
Toxome, 66
Trans fats, 126–27, 130, 153
Transgenerational effect, 65, 75
Treadmill exercise, 174–75
Tryptophan, 103, 110
Tufts University, 124
Tuna, 65, 133–34
Turmeric, 44, 140, 275
Tylenol, 73, 215

U
Ubiquinone, 138
UCLA, 181
University of Arizona, 156
University of California, Berkeley, 86
University of Cardiff, 145
University of Chicago, 99
University of Illinois, 156
University of Manchester, 271
University of Maryland Medical Center,
130
University of Massachusetts Medical School,
181
University of Miami, 151
University of Pennsylvania, 200
University of Pittsburgh, 156
University of Washington School of
Medicine, 156
Unsaturated fats, 126
USP certification, 269
Uterine cancer, 68

V
Variability, 25
Variable-intensity cardiovascular exercise
program, 160–61
Vascular dementia, 38
Vascular endothelial growth factor (VEGF),
159, 161
Vascular health, 149–53
Vegetables, 77–78, 124–25, 137, 139, 153
VEGF. *See* Vascular endothelial growth factor

Ventricles, 18
Verbal/auditory memory, 23
Video games, 238–39
Visual memory, 23–24
Vitamin B, 122–23, 124, 150, 152, 270–71
Vitamin B_1 (thiamin), 150, 152, 270
Vitamin B_2 (riboflavin), 150, 152, 270
Vitamin B_3 (niacin), 152, 270
Vitamin B_5 (pantothenic acid), 270
Vitamin B_6 (pyridoxine), 150, 152, 270
Vitamin B_{12} (cobalamin), 150, 152, 215, 270
Vitamin B_{12} deficiency test, 214
Vitamin C, 139, 152, 274
Vitamin D, 148, 267, 271–72
Vitamin E, 139, 273–74
Volunteering, 243–44
VO_2 maximum test, 164

W
Wake Forest University, 200
Walking, 157, 159–60
Walking backward, 228
Walnuts, 142–43
Water intake, 76–77
Wayne State University, 149
Wechsler Memory Scale, 216
Weizmann Institute of Science, 90
White matter hyperintensities (WMH),
149–50, 151
White tea, 142
Wine, red, 142, 274
Working memory, 24, 150, 200
World Health Organization (WHO), 273
Writing. *See* Journaling

X
Xanax (alprazolam), 109
Xenoestrogens, 68

Y
Yeast, 45, 75
Yogurt, 45, 121

Z
Zeaxanthin, 124
Zoloft, 96
Zuckerman, Enid, 219
Zuckerman, Mel, 219